Steering Group on the Microbiological Safety of Food

Annual Report 1994

LONDON: HMSO

ISBN 0 11 321939 3

The Steering Group on the Microbiological Safety of Food (SGMSF) was established in December 1990 with the following terms of reference:

"to identify through surveillance the need for action to ensure the microbiological safety of food."

The tasks remitted to the Steering Group by Ministers are detailed in its first[1] and second reports[2].

The Steering Group works in parallel with the Advisory Committee on the Microbiological Safety of Food. The Steering Group's relationship with the Advisory Committee is described in the Steering Group's first report.

Contents

FOREWORD

Our third Annual Report contains some encouraging news on Salmonella food poisoning although the general overall trend in the number of food poisoning notifications is still upwards. Only through carefully planned and co-ordinated national surveillance can we identify such trends and only through thorough analysis of outbreaks can we begin to tease out the important factors that contribute to food poisoning.

This year we have produced useful statistical guidance for those planning microbiological surveillance studies and our Compendium of Methods for Use in Microbiological Surveillance has been widely welcomed by food microbiologists both in the public and private sector. The results of a number of our studies are now beginning to appear including ready to eat meats, potential contamination sites in catering premises and items from self-service salad bars. Results of our survey of Salmonella contamination in raw chickens on retail sale will be published shortly.

The Steering Group has achieved a great deal since it was set up following the recommendation of the Richmond Committee. However, we must always strive to find more efficient ways of working and in the future the activities of the Steering Group will be merged with the Advisory Committee on the Microbiological Safety of Food. Co-ordinated microbiological surveillance will of course continue, but this will be the last Annual Report of the SGMSF. I should therefore like to express my very sincere thanks to all of the Members and Secretariat of the Steering Group and its Working Groups for all their hard work and for the spirit of co-operation which has greatly enhanced our ability to see and understand trends in microbiological food poisoning in the UK.

DR W H B DENNER
Chief Scientist (Food)
Chairman of the Steering Group on the
Microbiology Safety of Food

INTRODUCTION

1. This is the third report of the Steering Group on the Microbiological Safety of Food, covering the calendar year 1994.

2. During this period, the Steering Group met in plenary session on four occasions. In addition, there were a total of 20 meetings of its five Working Groups. The terms of reference of each of the Working Groups can be found in the Steering Group's first[1] and second[2] reports. The nomenclature used in classifying the various Steering Group surveillance studies is given at Appendix 6, paragraph 4.

3. Expenditure by the Ministry of Agriculture, Fisheries and Food and the Department of Health on surveillance activities undertaken under the aegis of the Steering Group amounted to £1,273,815 in 1994/95. A breakdown of this sum is given in Appendix 3.

Human Epidemiology Working Group

4.   The Human Epidemiology Working Group monitors trends in epidemiological data associated with foodborne illness in humans. Detailed information about these trends can be found in Appendix 4, Tables 1-5 and Figures 1-7. Food poisoning notifications are reports made to the Proper Officer by medical practitioners who suspect that illness may be caused by food, even though the cause of illness may not have been traced back to a food source or confirmed microbiologically. Laboratory reports of isolates refer to the number of laboratory isolations of certain pathogenic micro-organisms which are reported centrally to PHLS/CDSC. There is substantial under-reporting of both food poisoning notifications and laboratory isolates. Food poisoning notifications and reports of laboratory isolates are two sets of data which overlap but are not identical.

5.   Between 1993 and 1994 the number of notified cases of food poisoning increased in Northern Ireland by 5% and increased in Scotland by 26%. For the same period in England and Wales there was an increase of approximately 20% in the reports of formally notified cases plus cases ascertained by other means. Appendix 4, Table 1 and Figure 1.

6.   The most commonly reported laboratory isolates continue to be *Campylobacter* spp. and *Salmonella* spp. Campylobacteriosis continues to be the most commonly reported infectious intestinal disease in the UK. Appendix 4, Table 2 and Figure 2.

7.   Historically, notifications of food poisoning have followed a similar trend to the laboratory reports of *Salmonella* infection. However, in 1994 there was a slight overall decrease in UK laboratory reports of *Salmonella* compared with 1993.

8.   In England, Wales and Northern Ireland the overall number of laboratory reports of *Salmonella* infection to the PHLS/CDSC for 1994 was approximately 0.6% less than the 1993 total. Within this total the number of reports of *Salmonella enteritidis* 'phage type 4 decreased by 20% in England and Wales. In Scotland, there was approximately a 2% increase in *Salmonella* infections reported to SCIEH although the number of reports of *Salmonella enteritidis* 'phage type 4 decreased by about 10%. Appendix 4, Table 3 and Figures 3-5.

9.   In England and Wales *Salmonella typhimurium* DT104 is the second most frequently reported *Salmonella* in humans after *Salmonella enteritidis* 'phage type 4. In 1994 there were 2,848 laboratory reports of *Salmonella typhimurium* DT104 of which 2,116 were resistant to ampicillin, chloramphenicol, streptomycin, sulphonamides and tetracyclines (R-type ACSSuT). This compares with 1,208 reports of multi-resistant isolates in 1993. This represents an increase of 75% on 1993 figures.

10.   In May a joint meeting was held with the Farm Animals and Abattoirs Surveillance Working Group. The purpose was to discuss the rise in *Salmonella typhimurium* DT104 infection in animals and humans. As a result of the discussion it was agreed that both groups would keep the epidemiological data under review whilst awaiting the results of various studies being undertaken.

11.   The number of cases of human listeriosis in the UK continues to be at a low level compared with the period 1987-1989. There were 102 confirmed cases in England and Wales in 1993 and 112 in 1994 (provisional data). In Scotland there were 12 cases in 1993 and 12 in 1994. In Northern Ireland 1 case was reported in 1994 (provisional data) and 4 cases in 1993. Appendix 4 Table 4 and Figure 6.

12.   The number of isolates of verocytotoxin-producing *Escherichia coli* O157 in England and Wales increased from 385 in 1993 to 411 in 1994. In Scotland, the number of laboratory reports of faecal isolates rose from 119 in 1993 to 242 in 1994. Reporting of this pathogen began in 1982 with

the peak year so far in Scotland being 1994. In England and Wales the peak year so far was 1992 with 470 laboratory reports of faecal isolates. The rate of infection per 100,000 population continues to be highest in Scotland compared with the rest of the UK. Appendix 4, Table 5 and Figure 7. In 1994 outbreaks were reported in Scotland associated with burger meat, pasteurised milk and cheese made from raw milk.

13.   The current work of the Human Epidemiology Working Group includes the Study of Infectious Intestinal Disease (IID) in England which started in July 1993. The study is a collaborative venture between the Medical Research Council Epidemiology and Medical Care Unit, the Public Health Laboratory Service, the London School of Hygiene and Tropical Medicine and the Department of Health. The study will take place over three years in 70 General Practices of the MRC General Practice Framework. Practices have been selected to be representative of general practices in England in terms of location, size of practice, urban or rural location, and Jarman deprivation score. The components of the study are:

- a population cohort study which will estimate the incidence and aetiology of IID in the general population.

- a GP based case-control study of IID cases presenting to GPs.

- an enumeration study to estimate the incidence of IID presenting to GPs and the proportion of samples routinely sent for microbiological examination.

- a study of the socio-economic costs of IID.

14.   The study is progressing satisfactorily and almost all practices have been recruited. Field and laboratory work is expected to be completed in 1996.

15.   In conjunction with the Retail, Catering and Consumer Surveillance Working Group, a sub-group was set up to investigate the need for studies of consumer food handling practices. Further details are given in paragraph 59.

16.   A project proposal on the prevalence of verocytotoxin-producing *Escherichia coli* O157 in the Sheffield area was considered by the Steering Group and will be funded by the Department of Health. The aim of this two year study is to examine the prevalence of verocytotoxin-producing *E.coli* O157 in a), faecal swabs from farm animals at slaughter b), a variety of foodstuffs at retail outlets and c), in stool samples from humans with acute uncomplicated diarrhoea.

Farm Animals and Abattoir Surveillance Working Group

17.   The Farm Animals and Abbattoir Surveillance Working Group has been monitoring trends in the epidemiological data associated with zoonotic infections in animals and poultry. Information regarding these trends is summarised in Appendix 5, Tables 1-14.

18.   Cattle: Reported incidents of *Salmonella* infection in cattle increased during 1994 due largely to the continuing rise in the incidence of *Salmonella typhimurium* DT 104 (Appendix 5, Table 1 and 6). This is now the predominant *Salmonella typhimurium* phage type in cattle. Epidemiological investigations are underway (see Case Control Study in later paragraphs).

19.   Sheep: *Salmonella* incidents reported from sheep rose in 1994 though the rise was not significant and the total number of reported incidents remain at the levels seen in the past 10 years. However, as with cattle and pigs, there was a sharp rise in reported incidents of *Salmonella typhimurium* DT 104 (Appendix 5, Table 2 and 7).

20.   Pigs: *Salmonella derby* and *Salmonella typhimurium* were the most frequently reported serotypes from pigs. There was a sharp rise in the number of *Salmonella typhimurium* DT104 incidents reported in 1994 (Appendix 5, Table 3 and 8).

21.   Poultry: There was a further fall in reported incidents of *Salmonella enteritidis* and *Salmonella typhimurium* from poultry (Appendix 5, Table 4 and 5). This is most marked in broilers and broiler breeders and hopefully reflects the medium term effects of Government and industry measures taken to control infection with these two serotypes.

22.   Animal feedingstuffs: The 1992 report of the Expert Group on Animal Feedingstuffs, chaired by Professor Eric Lamming, recommended that the Ministry should try to improve the information it collected on *Salmonella* in animal feedingstuffs. This recommendation was implemented in September 1992 by asking all laboratories testing samples of animal feedingstuffs to provide the Ministry with enhanced information. The results of this monitoring are summarised in Appendix 5, Table 10. The table shows the large number of tests being performed on animal feedingstuffs as a result of MAFF/Industry Codes of Practice for the control of *Salmonella*, producing comprehensive information on the microbiological status of feedingstuffs. The results suggest that the microbiological status of processed animal proteins arriving at compounders for feedingstuffs use may have increased during 1994, although the overall contamination rates of finished compounds is similar to 1993.

23.   On 1 January 1993, the Animal By-Products Order 1992 came into effect, implementing the provisions of Directive 90/667/EEC on the disposal and processing of animal waste. Under this Order, animal by-products have to be disposed of to specified outlets including approved or registered rendering, petfood, pharmaceutical or technical plants, or to knackers, hunt kennels and certain other outlets. They can also be buried or incinerated.

24.   Rendering premises must register under the Processed Animal Protein Order 1989. This Order requires processors to submit samples of processed animal protein to an approved laboratory for *Salmonella* testing on each day that product leaves their premises. If tests prove positive, no product may leave the premises for incorporation into animal or poultry feedingstuffs unless certain conditions specified in the Order are complied with. In addition, Ministry staff carry out quarterly inspections of all registered premises and sample 20 day's production for *Salmonella* through the year. Appendix 5, Table 12 shows how the microbiological status of processed animal protein has improved since 1988, with only 2.5 per cent of the samples taken in the course of official testing during 1994 being contaminated with *Salmonella*. The contamination rate was slightly higher than 1993. This may be

due, in part, to the temporary interference caused by plant alterations as a result of the new rendering conditions required under Commission Decision 94/382/EEC. The consequences of a fire at a large rendering premises also caused one persistent contamination incident.

Survey of *E. coli* O157:H7 in bovine faeces

25.   A survey of *E. coli* O157:H7 carriage rates in live cattle based on the screening of all bovine faeces samples submitted to MAFF Veterinary Investigation Centres in England and Wales and to the Veterinary Investigation Service of the Scottish Agricultural Colleges commenced in June 1994. The survey will run for 12 consecutive months over which period it is expected 9,000 samples will be examined. Information will additionally be collected on the geographical location, age and breed type of positive animals as well as the reason samples were presented for examination. At 31 December 1994, 3,602 samples had been examined from 2,644 herds of which 24 samples were positive for *E. coli* O157:H7.

Survey of *E. coli* O157:H7 carriage rates on beef carcases

26.   A survey of *E. coli* O157:H7 carriages rates on beef carcases leaving abattoirs in the United Kingdom commenced on 1 September and will run for 12 consecutive months. During the period of the survey, veterinary staff from the various Agriculture Departments will visit 198 abattoirs, collect samples from 4,460 beef carcases and examine them for *E. coli* O157:H7. At 31 December 1994, 1,360 samples had been collected of which 3 were positive for *E. coli* O157:H7.

Case control study of *Salmonella typhimurium* DT 104 in cattle

27.   The incidence of a strain of *Salmonella typhimurium* DT 104 exhibiting chromosomal resistance to ampicillin, chloramphenicol, streptomycin, sulphonamides and tetracycline (R - ACSSuT) is rising in humans and a number of farmed animal species, particularly cattle, in Great Britain. Until 1985, *Salmonella typhimurium* DT 104 was restricted to cattle and its incidence was low based on notifications made under the Zoonoses Order 1975. Since then the number of incidents reported from cattle has increased, most of the increase being due to the multi-resistant strain. It is now the most common *Salmonella typhimurium* reported from cattle.

28.   Initial epidemiological investigations into the human outbreak suggest that the epidemiology of *Salmonella typhimurium* DT 104 is more complex than is normal for *Salmonella* infections and that no single contaminated foodstuff is responsible for human infection. A number of cases have occurred in people caring for livestock, particularly calves, indicating that there is an occupational health risk for farm staff. Initial investigations into the disease in cattle suggest an equally complex picture in cattle and contaminated feedingstuffs, movement of livestock, wild birds and the spreading of sewage sludge on agricultural land have all been implicated in recent outbreaks of disease.

29.   Little is known about potential sources of infection in other species. Initial reports suggest that that the organism is more pathogenic for cattle than many other salmonellas with higher than normal mortality rate in all ages of livestock.

30.   High priority is attached to investigations into the causes of multi-resistant *Salmonella typhimurium* DT 104 incidents in agricultural livestock and poultry, the aim being to understand the epidemiology of infection so as to devise appropriate control strategies. This is being achieved by a specific Case Control study in cattle and an accelerated programme of visits to incidents in pigs, sheep

and domestic fowl reported under the Zoonoses Order 1989.

31.   In the period August 1994 to June 1995, MAFF veterinary staff will visit 200 herds from which incidents of *Salmonella typhimurium* DT 104 infection have been reported and 200 "control" herds with no previous history of *Salmonella* infection.   The purpose of these visits will be two fold:

   (a)   to advise on disease control and protection of farm workers;

   (b)   to collect data for the case control study.

Information will be collected on a range of risk factors thought likely to influence the introduction and spread of disease on farms.   It is hoped that when analysed, the information will assist in devising appropriate control strategies.

Survey of *Salmonella* contamination in cereals used in animal feedingstuffs

32.   In the past four years, there has been growing concern at the number of isolations of *Salmonella* spp. from cereal feed ingredients used in animal feedingstuffs.   Based on numerator and denominator data provided by laboratories testing raw material and finished animal feeds under MAFF Codes of Practice for the Control of *Salmonella* in Animal Feedingstuffs, annual *Salmonella* contamination rates in finished feeds for ruminants, pigs and poultry ranged from 2.1% - 4.7% in 1993. While these contamination rates might be regarded as low and compare favourably with data from other European Union Member States, cereal raw ingredients comprise in excess of 90% of finished feed rations and can therefore act as an important route by which *Salmonella* spp may enter the food chain.

33.   At present, all isolations of *Salmonella enteritidis* and *Salmonella typhimurium* reported from feed mills are investigated by the MAFF State Veterinary Service, a comprehensive microbiological audit of compounding premises being undertaken to try to identify where contamination is taking place so that advice on control can be given.   However, the reason for this apparent increase remains unclear and it was felt important to determine (a) the true rate of contamination and (b) the factors leading to contamination so that these could be better understood and consequently minimised.   To this end, a survey of *Salmonella* contamination in cereals delivered to compounder's premises is being undertaken.   This will be supplemented by a longitudinal study of contamination on farms/storage facilities to identify the management factors associated with contamination and the risk of persistent or future discrete occurrences.

34.   In the period 1 September - 31 December 1994, 2,365 samples of whole grain cereals (wheat, barley and oats) were collected from consignments arriving at 41 feedmills in Great Britain and examined for *Salmonella* spp. at MAFF veterinary laboratories. Only 5 samples were found to be contaminated with *Salmonella*.

Food Processing Surveillance Working Group

Membership

35.   Towards the end of 1994, Miss Claire Cunningham of LACOTS (Local Authority Co-ordinating Body on Food and Trading Standards) was invited to become a member of the Food Processing Working Group.

National Study of Ready to Eat Meats and Meat Products: Part 1

36.   Sampling for the first part of the National Study of ready to eat meats and meat products (RTE) began in November 1993. The study was limited to those RTE processors that cooked and further processed products on the same premises. Although the majority of samples had been collected by the scheduled finish date of March 1994, difficulties in the identification of suitable paté processors meant that the last few samples were not taken until July 1994. In all, 48 ham processors and 53 pork pie processors were visited. Despite the fact that the criteria for the inclusion of paté processors were redefined, only 16 suitable establishments were identified and visited. However, statistical analysis of the paté results, showed that sufficient numbers had been taken to allow comparisons to be made with the other two products.

37.   The RTE Study involved 22 samplers (predominantly Environmental Health Department personnel) with 8 laboratories carrying out microbiological and chemical analyses of the surveillance samples. Samplers were asked when visiting a processor to take samples at 3 distinct stages of production; immediately after cooking, after a further processing stage (e.g. slicing, jellying, etc.) and from the final holding store prior to distribution. In all, 352 samples were taken from 122 products with a total of 2,128 analyses (1,888 microbiological and 240 chemical) being carried out.

38.   *Listeria monocytogenes* was isolated from 8 (6.7%) of the 119 products, 6 hams, 1 paté and 1 pork pie. *Listeria monocytogenes* enumeration was carried out on the final hold samples and in the one incidence where a count was obtained, from a final hold ham sample, the level was low, (less than 20 organisms per gram). The enumeration of *Staphylococcus aureus* was carried out on the final hold samples with 5 of the 119 samples tested (4.2%) providing counts. Four of these were from ham samples and 1 from a pork pie and all were at a level of less than 100 organisms per gram. *Salmonella* spp. or *Campylobacter* spp. were not isolated from any of the samples examined. A summary of the total viable counts and Enterobacteriaceae levels found in the 3 products is given in Table 1. A report on Part I of the study has been produced and accepted by the Food Processing Working Group and will be published in the near future.

National Study of Ready to Eat Meats and Meat Products: Part 2

39.   The preparation of Part 2 of the National Study of ready to eat meats and meat products was completed by the end of 1994. This study looked at four product types: cured, cooked pork (whole muscle); cured, cooked, comminuted meat; poultry (whole muscle); and corned beef and was aimed at secondary processors of RTE meats. These were defined as processors that, having brought in the bulk product ready cooked, proceeded to slice and pack it prior to distribution. Samples were analysed microbiologically for the presence/absence of: *Listeria* spp., *Listeria monocytogenes*, *Salmonella* spp., *Campylobacter* spp. and *Escherichia coli* O157:H7. Additionally the following organisms were be tested quantitatively: Total Viable Count, Total Enterobacteriaceae, *Listeria monocytogenes*, *Staphylococcus aureus* and *Clostridium perfringens*. Sampling for Part 2 of the National Study took

place between January and March 1995. A Report will be published later in the year.

Sampler Training

40.   During 1994 an attempt was made to increase the numbers of samplers available for use in the studies of the Food Processing Working Group. This was felt to be of particular importance, in view of the difficulties that were encountered identifying sufficient suitable processors in the final pilot study for the RTE study and the National Study Part 1. Following a request to Food Liaison Groups in England and Wales at the end of 1993 approximately 80 nominations for samplers were obtained. Initially, 2 sampler training days were held at the start of 1994 with the 15 samplers who attended being included in the National Study Part 1. In August and September a further 59 samplers attended 5 training days and this brought the total number of samplers to just over 100. Samplers commented that the training days were of significant benefit, particularly regarding aseptic techniques. It is the intention that only trained samplers will be used in the studies of the Food Processing Working Group.

41.   Although there is generally a good geographical distribution of samplers throughout England and Wales, the Scientific Secretariat of the Food Processing Working Group will endeavour to recruit samplers from the few areas that are not covered during 1995. With the number of samplers now available to the Food Processing Working Group it is anticipated that many of the difficulties that were encountered during the National Study Part 1 have now been overcome and that future studies will proceed much more smoothly.

Quality Assessment Scheme

42.   In the Autumn of 1993, all laboratories possessing NAMAS (National Measurement and Accreditation Service) accreditation for the microbiological analysis of food and food products were asked if they wished to be considered to receive samples from the surveillance studies of the FPWG. Six ADAS food laboratories, who were well advanced in the appropriate accreditation, were also approached. Those laboratories willing to receive samples have been participating since November 1993 in a quality assessment scheme. This was set up to allow the FPWG to assess how well laboratories could measure the contamination of foods, by defined organisms, using the microbiological methods laid down. Samples are sent to laboratories bimonthly and are composed of a base matrix (freeze dried minced beef or chicken) inoculated with a range of bacteria. Approximately 30 laboratories took part and satisfactory performance is required for a laboratory to remain in the scheme and be able to receive surveillance samples. Following unsatisfactory performance after one year's involvement, two laboratories (who had not received surveillance samples) have been removed from the scheme. One laboratory has been given a warning that improvement in their performance is required before they receive any samples. More laboratories will be recruited to the scheme as the need arises.

Surveillance of Canneries

43.   Following a request from the Steering Group to investigate canning, the Campden and Chorleywood Food Research Association were commissioned by the Food Processing Working Group to conduct a survey so that an objective view could be formed on the extent of risks posed to the consumer of canned foods. The survey was designed to determine the level of technical expertise

available in a cannery, together with the extent to which this expertise was applied to the manufacturing process, and, as such, involved no microbiological sampling. The survey began in the autumn of 1994 and was completed in February 1995. A total of 40 canneries in the UK, of which the majority are small operations, were visited. A report on the canneries survey is expected to be published later in the year.

Targeting Study of Warm Water Prawns

44.   Preparation for a Targeting Study of UK processors of warm water prawns was completed by December 1994. These processors, which are defined as those that import raw product prior to heat treatment in the UK, are relatively few in number (less than 10) and it is the intention that each participating processor will be visited on three occasions. Samples will be analysed microbiologically for the presence/absence of: *Listeria* spp., *Listeria monocytogenes*, *Salmonella* spp., *Campylobacter* spp., *Aeromonas hydrophila*, *Vibrio parahaemolyticus* and *Vibrio* spp.. Additionally, the following will be tested for quantitatively: Total Viable Count, Total Enterobacteriaceae, *Listeria monocytogenes*, *Staphylococcus aureus*, *Escherchia coli* and *Vibrio parahaemolyticus*. Sampling began in March 1995 and will continue until sufficient numbers of samples have been taken. A report on the study of warm water prawns is expected to be published later in the year.

45.   Following a request from the Steering Group, the Targeting Study has been adapted to include imported, cooked, warm water prawns, i.e. those that are processed abroad and enter the UK in a ready to eat state. This will allow a comparison to be made between warm water prawns processed in the UK and abroad. Sampling for this part of the study began in March 1995 and will continue until sufficient numbers of samples have been taken.

Study of Cooked, Chilled, Plain Chicken

46.   During 1994 work has continued on the protocols for a study of cooked, chilled, plain chicken. The protocols were discussed by the Food Processing Working Group and the Retail, Catering and Consumer Surveillance Working Group. A decision on the protocols will be made at a later date.

Table 1: Summary of Total Viable Count and Enterobacteriaceae Results from the RTE National Study Part I

1a: Paté

$\log_{10}$ cfu/g	Cook Stage		Slice/Jellying Stage		Final Hold Stage	
<1.00	2	(15)*	1	(10)	1	(13)
1.00-1.99	0	(0)	2	(3)	2	(1)
2.00-2.99	8	(1)	3	(0)	5	(2)
3.00-3.99	5	(0)	4	(0)	2	(0)
4.00-4.99	0	(0)	3	(0)	3	(0)
5.00-5.99	0	(0)	0	(0)	0	(0)
>6.00	1	(0)	0	(0)	3	(0)

1b: Pork Pie

$\log_{10}$ cfu/g	Cook Stage		Slice/Jellying Stage		Final Hold Stage	
<1.00	28	(53)	30	(50)	19	(53)
1.00-1.99	14	(0)	12	(0)	16	(0)
2.00-2.99	9	(1)	6	(2)	14	(0)
3.00-3.99	2	(0)	3	(0)	3	(0)
4.00-4.99	1	(0)	2	(1)	1	(1)
5.00-5.99	0	(0)	0	(0)	1	(0)
>6.00	0	(0)	0	(0)	1	(1)

1c: Ham

$\log_{10}$ cfu/g	Cook Stage		Slice/Jellying Stage		Final Hold Stage	
<1.00	23	(48)	4	(42)	3	(43)
1.00-1.99	15	(0)	9	(3)	4	(1)
2.00-2.99	7	(0)	11	(2)	19	(3)
3.00-3.99	2	(0)	13	(0)	11	(2)
4.00-4.99	1	(0)	10	(1)	10	(0)
5.00-5.99	0	(0)	1	(0)	0	(0)
>6.00	0	(0)	0	(0)	2	(0)

* Figures in brackets relate to the Enterobacteriaceae results.

Retail, Catering and Consumer Surveillance Working Group

47.   During the course of the year, a number of studies were started and are in various stages of completion. These were:

Project on Potential Contamination Sites in Catering Premises

48.   A targeting study of contamination of food contact and hand contact surfaces in catering premises started in April 1994. The interest in food contact surfaces arose from a concern that they may provide a source of cross contamination of food, which may be a contributory factor in causing foodborne illness. In addition there was little published information on either the survival of micro-organisms on different food contact surfaces or the potential for their transfer to food.

49.   The Working Group had earlier conducted a pilot study to test possible study methods and to indicate suitable target areas. A small project was also commissioned to establish a methodology for the recovery of *Campylobacter*, which was completed satisfactorily and its results are to be published in the International Journal of Food Microbiology. Following these projects, the Steering Group agreed that a targeting study should be carried out.

50.   The study started in April 1994 with the aim of obtaining data about levels of contamination on food contact and hand contact surfaces . The study was confined to catering premises where both raw and cooked foods were handled. The Environmental Health Departments and Public Health Laboratories in the Exeter and Sheffield areas conducted this study.

51.   The field work has been completed and the results are currently being analysed. The report will be presented to the Steering Group which will consider the need for further studies. The results will be published in 1995.

Study on Bacteriological Examination of Salad Items and Hors d'Oeuvres from Self-Service Salad Bars

52.   A targeting study of the bacteriological status of salad items and hors d'oeuvres in self-service salad bars in restaurants started in June 1994. The Working Group's interest arose from a concern that the microbiological safety of the food could be compromised where customers have unsupervised access to foods. Following a pilot study to test practical feasibility and identify suitable target areas, the Steering Group agreed that a targeting study should be carried out looking specifically at restaurant outlets.

53.   The study began in June 1994. Samples were taken from a range of salad products including shellfish, chicken, sliced meats, smoked fish, rice, pasta, mayonnaise and mayonnaise-based mixed salads. The analysis looked for the presence and in some cases, the numbers of a range of micro-organisms. Premises sampled in the study included pubs, restaurants, hotel restaurants and take-away and fast food restaurants. After a competitive tendering exercise, the study was undertaken by Food Liaison Groups in Cheshire, Cleveland, Devon, Kent and South Yorkshire.

54.   The field work has been completed and the results are being analysed. The results are expected to be published in 1995.

Survey of *Salmonella* Contamination in UK Produced Raw Chicken

55.   A survey of *Salmonella* contamination in UK produced raw chickens on retail sale was undertaken by the Working Group in response to a request from the Advisory Committee on the Microbiological Safety of Food. The study had a secondary aim to examine the comparability of previous and current *Salmonella* detection methods in order to provide a basis for comparability of results between past, present and future studies. The study was supplemented by a separate study of Scottish chickens. The results will be published in 1995.

Surveillance of the Microbiological Safety of Raw (Green Top) Cow's Milk on Retail Sale

56.   A survey of the microbiological quality of raw (green top) cow's milk on retail sale was agreed by the Steering Group and started early in 1995.

Other Projects/Activities

57.   The Working Group also commented upon a number of research proposals which had been received by the Department of Health. Support was given to a study of microbial colonisation and survival on surfaces being undertaken by King's College (London). This followed consideration by the Working Group of a number of reports on the relative merits of wooden and plastic chopping boards.

58.   The study of cooked chicken to be undertaken in conjunction with the Food Processing Working Group has been deferred until the summer of 1995.

59.   In order to explore possibilities for surveillance in the domestic sphere, a symposium was held (jointly with the Human Epidemiology Working Group) in March. The Steering Group confirmed the need for further information. Areas of particular interest were behaviour in the home, hygiene, the data collected during investigations of outbreaks of food poisoning, and labelling. A sub-group has been set up to consider these issues further.

60.   During the year steps were taken to improve co-ordination of Steering Group work and other studies undertaken by local authorities, including their participation in the Local Authority Co-ordinating Body on Food and Trading Standards (LACOTS) Food Sampling Programme. Links had been reinforced between the Steering Group and LACOTS with the aim of keeping both sides fully informed of work being planned and undertaken. In addition, it was also agreed that, in order to aid the comparison of results, studies undertaken by LACOTS would, where appropriate, use methods endorsed by the Steering Group. The Working Group exchanges with LACOTS details of studies proposed and takes these into account when considering its programme of work.

Research Working Group

61.   The Working Group has continued to comment on and advise on study protocols submitted by the other Working Groups as mentioned in their sections of this report. In addition, the Working Group produced guidelines on surveillance study protocols for use by the other Working Groups.

Guidelines on Surveillance Study Protocols

62.   The guidelines include guidance already given on an ad hoc basis on microbiological methods, statistics and laboratory accreditation, and include advice on new topics such as sampling methods and the archiving of isolates and clinical samples. These guidelines are available on request to external organisations carrying out surveillance, such as Environmental Health Departments and the Public Health Laboratory Service.

Methods for use in Microbiological Surveillance

63.   In June, the Steering Group published a compendium of microbiological methods, Methods for Use in Microbiological Surveillance, which had been compiled by the Working Group. The aim of this compendium was to encourage organisations which undertake microbiological surveillance to use the same methods in order to improve the consistency of the data produced, thereby allowing valid scientific comparisons to be made. The compendium was distributed widely to relevant organisations including Environmental Health Departments, the Public Health Laboratory Service, National Health Service and other laboratories undertaking the microbiological analysis of food, clinical and environmental samples, food research associations, professional bodies and trade associations. It is intended that the compendium will be updated as necessary to incorporate new methods and changes in existing methods.

Workshop on Foodborne Viral Infections

64.   A workshop on foodborne viral infections was held in October. The Advisory Committee on the Microbiological Safety of Food had previously considered a literature review of foodborne viruses and had asked the Steering Group for a view on the adequacy of epidemiological investigation of outbreaks of viral foodborne disease. The Steering Group had concluded that there was a need for research into improved detection methods. Subsequently, the Advisory Committee and Steering Group had agreed that a joint workshop would be a useful means of clarifying the current state of knowledge about foodborne viruses and considering opportunities and priorities for research.

65.   Speakers at the Workshop included leading authorities on foodborne viral infection from academia, the National Health Service, the Public Health Laboratory Service, the travel industry, MAFF and the US Centers for Disease Control and Prevention.

66.   The workshop reached a consensus view that small round structured viruses (SRSVs) were the priority group and that specific areas for further work were: improved detection methods for SRSVs in foods; molecular methods for epidemiological surveillance; data on the survival of viruses in foods; and improved methods for depuration and surveillance of shellfish, especially bivalve molluscs. The Research Working Group is considering the options for taking these areas forward.

Steering Group on the Microbiological Safety of Food

List of members at the end of the period under report

<u>Chairman</u>

Dr W H B Denner	- MAFF, Chief Scientist (Food)

<u>Members</u>

Dr G Jones (Deputy Chairman)	- DH, Head of Health Aspects of the Environment and Food Medical Division
Dr A C Baird-Parker	- Head of Microbiology, Unilever Research
Dr C Bartlett	- Director CDSC, PHLS
Dr J R Bell	- MAFF, Head of Food Science Division II
Mr B Bridges	- DH, Under Secretary, Health Aspects of the Environment and Food Administrative Division
Dr R J Cawthorne	- MAFF, Head of Animal Health (Zoonoses) Division
Mr R Cunningham	- DH, Assistant Secretary, Health Aspects of the Environment and Food Administrative Division
Dr M Cooke	- Deputy Director, PHLS
Mr K J Dale	- MAFF Head of Quality and Microbiology Unit, Food Science Division II
Mr E C Davison	- SOAFD, Assistant Secretary, Animal Health and Food Safety Division (until August 1994)
Mr B H B Dickinson	- MAFF, Under Secretary, Food Safety Group
Professor C Easmon	- British Post Graduate Medical Federation
Dr P Fine	- London School of Hygiene and Tropical Medicine
Mr M T Haddon	- MAFF, Under Secretary, Animal Health Veterinary Group
Dr D Harper	- DH, Health Aspects of the Environment and Food Medical Division
Mr I C Henderson	- DANI, Assistant Secretary
Dr M Hinton	- University of Bristol (from April 1994)
Mr E W Kingcott	- DH, Chief Environmental Health Officer, Health Aspects of the Environment and Food Medical Division
Mr D MacDonald	- SOAFD, Chief Food and Dairy Officer (from August 1994)
Dr A MacLeod	- SOHHD, Senior Medical Officer (until October 1994)
Dr P Madden	- SOHHD, Senior Medical Officer (from October 1994)
Dr E Mitchell	- DHSS(NI), Senior Medical Officer
Miss J Morris	- Safeway Stores plc
Mrs S Payne	- Consumer
Mr E Ramsden	- Chief Environmental Health Officer, Swansea
Dr T A Roberts	- Institute of Food Research
Dr R Skinner	- DH, Principal Medical Officer, Health Aspects of the Environment and Food Medical Division
Professor I M Smith	- Royal Veterinary College (until March 1994)
Mr M Verstringhe	- Chairman, Catering and Allied Services Ltd.

<u>Secretariat</u>

Mr C R Mylchreest	- MAFF, Microbiological Safety of Food Division
Dr R T Mitchell	- MAFF, Food Science Division II
Mrs S Gordon Brown	- DH, Health Aspects of the Environment and Food Administrative Division
Dr L Robinson	- DH, Health Aspects of the Environment and Food Medical Division
Dr V King	- DH, Health Aspects of the Environment and Food Medical Division
Mr E Bates	- MAFF, Microbiological Safety of Food Division

Human Epidemiology Working Group

Chairman

Dr R Skinner	- DH, Principal Medical Officer, Health Aspects of the Environment and Food Medical Division

Members

Dr B Bannister	- Coppett's Wood Hospital
Dr R J Cawthorne	- MAFF, Head of Animal Health (Zoonoses) Division
Dr J Cowden	- PHLS, CDSC
Professor R Feldman	- London Hospital Medical College
Mr C Lister	- DH, Health Aspects of the Environment and Food Administrative Division
Dr A MacLeod	- SOHHD, Senior Medical Officer (until October 1994)
Dr P Madden	- SOHHD, Senior Medical Officer (from October 1994)
Dr E Mitchell	- Department of Health and Social Services (Northern Ireland)
Mrs A M Pickering	- MAFF, Head of Microbiological Safety of Food Division
Mr W Reilly	- Scottish Centre for Infection and Environmental Health
Dr B Rowe	- PHLS, Director of the Laboratory of Enteric Pathogens

Secretariat

Mrs S Gordon Brown	- DH, Health Aspects of the Environment and Food Administrative Division
Dr V King	- DH, Health Aspects of the Environment and Food Medical Division
Mr K Borowski	- DH, Health Aspects of the Environment and Food Administrative Division

Farm Animals and Abattoir Surveillance Working Group

Chairman

Dr R J Cawthorne	- MAFF, Head of Animal Health (Zoonoses) Division

Members

Mr T E D Eddy	- MAFF, Head of Animal Health (Disease Control) Division
Dr M Hinton	- University of Bristol
Dr T M Humphrey	- Public Health Laboratory Service
Dr A M Johnston	- Royal Veterinary College
Dr R M McCracken	- DANI, Deputy Chief Veterinary Officer
Mr T Murray	- DH, Health Aspects of the Environment and Food Administrative Division
Dr R Skinner	- DH, Principal Medical Officer, Health Aspects of the Environment and Food Medical Division
Professor I M Smith	- Royal Veterinary College
Mr J W Wilesmith	- MAFF, Central Veterinary Laboratory
Dr D Williams	BOCM Silcock Laboratory

Secretariat

Mr D Bower	- MAFF, Animal Health (Zoonoses) Division
Mr E Bates	- MAFF, Microbiological Safety of Food Division

Food Processing Surveillance Working Group

Chairman
Mr K J Dale   - MAFF Head of Quality and Microbiology Unit, Food Science Division II

Members
Mr D Atherton   - Princes Ltd.
Dr A C Baird-Parker   - Unilever Research
Mr B M Bruce   - Christian Salveson Food Services Ltd.
Mr B Bradley   - DH, Health Aspects of the Environment and Food Medical Division
Ms C Cunningham   - LACOTS (from August 1994)
Ms C Endacott-Palmer   - Van den Bergh Foods Ltd.
Mr A Hacking   - ADAS, Wales
Mr J Harris   - MAFF, State Veterinary Service
Mr E Kingcott   - Chief Environmental Health Officer, Department of Health
Mr D MacDonald   - Scottish Office Agriculture and Fisheries Department
Dr A Moore   - ADAS
Mr C Morrison   - UB Ross-Youngs Ltd.
Dr M Patterson   - DANI, Food Microbiology Research Division
Mrs L Pugh   - Wellingborough Environmental Health Department
Mr D Smith   - Master Food Europe

Secretariat
Dr R T Mitchell   - MAFF, Food Science Division II (Chairman from 1 January 1995)
Dr J P Back   - MAFF, Food Science Division II
Mr E Bates   - MAFF, Microbiological Safety of Food Division
Miss K J Harmon   - MAFF, Microbiological Safety of Food Division

Retail, Catering and Consumer Surveillance Working Group

Chairman
Mr E Kingcott   - DH, Chief Environmental Health Officer

Members
Dr L Ackerley   - Hygiene Audit Systems
Miss H Asmah   - Tesco Stores plc
Dr J P Back   - MAFF, Food Science Division II
Dr J E L Corry   - Bristol University, Department of Veterinary Medicines
Mr K J Dale   - MAFF, Head of Quality and Microbiology Unit, Food Science Division II
Mr W P Davidson   - Director of Environmental Health, Stewarty District Council
Dr M Gasson   - Institute of Food Research (IFR), Norwich Laboratory
Dr J de Louvois   - PHLS, CDSC
Mr G McCurdy   - Dept. of Environment Northern Ireland
Mr T Miller   - Commercial Development Manager, Whitbread PLC
Mr C R Mylchreest   - MAFF, Microbiological Safety of Food Division
Mr M Norman   - Wm Low & Co. plc
Mrs S Payne   - Consumer
Mr M Verstringhe   - Catering and Allied Services
Dr S Walker   - Campden Food and Drink Research Association (CFDRA)

Secretariat
Mr B Bradley   - DH, Health Aspects of the Environment and Food Medical Division
Mrs S Gordon Brown   - DH, Health Aspects of the Environment and Food Administrative Division
Mr K Borowski   - DH, Health Aspects of the Environment and Food Administrative Division

Research Working Group

Chairman

Dr D Harper   - DH, Health Aspects of the Environment and Food Medical Division

Members

Dr A C Baird-Parker   - Unilever Research
Dr E O Caul   - Bristol Public Health Laboratory, Public Health Laboratory Service
Dr I Farrell   - Birmingham Public Health Laboratory, Public Health Laboratory Service
Dr V King   - DH, Health Aspects of the Environment and Food Medical Division
Dr J P Back   - MAFF, Food Science Division II
Dr T A Roberts   - Institute of Food Research
Dr M Stringer   - Campden Food and Drink Research Association
Dr C Wray   - Central Veterinary Laboratory

Secretariat

Mr B Bradley   - DH, Health Aspects of the Environment and Food Medical Division
Mr G M Robb   - DH, Health Aspects of the Environment and Food Administrative Division
Mr K Borowski   - DH, Health Aspects of the Environment and Food Administrative Division

Domestic Practices Sub-Group

Chairman

Mr E Kingcott   - DH, Chief Environmental Health Officer

Members

Dr L Ackerley   - Hygiene Audit Systems
Mrs W Browne   - Medical Research Council, Wolfson Institute of Preventative Medicine
Dr J Cowden   - PHLS, CDSC
Dr J Holland   - Social Sciences Research Unit, Institute of Education, University of London
Mr M Hudson   - Centre for Applied Microbiology and Research (CAMR)
Mr P Martin   - DH, Health Aspects of the Environment and Food Administrative Division
Mr M D Norman   - Wm Low & Co plc
Mrs S Payne   - Consumer
Ms W Spence   - J Sainsbury plc

Secretariat

Mr B Bradley   - DH, Health Aspects of the Environment and Food Medical Division
Mrs S Gordon Brown   - DH, Health Aspects of the Environment and Food Administrative Division
Mr K Borowski   - DH, Health Aspects of the Environment and Food Administrative Division

Register of Members' Interests

Non-Governmental members are appointed to the Steering Group for the expertise they have gained in their professional involvement in the area of the microbiological safety of food, and not because of their employment or involvement in any given organisation. Group members are reminded at the start of each meeting to declare any interest in the matters to be discussed. The Chairman may then, at his or her discretion, limit the participation of a member in a discussion. Ministers consider it important that the Group's advice should not be subject to suspicion of bias on the grounds of undeclared commercial interest.

REGISTER OF MEMBERS' INTERESTS

MEMBER	PERSONAL INTERESTS		NON-PERSONAL INTERESTS	
	Name of Company	Nature of Interest	Name of Company	Nature of Interest
Dr A Baird-Parker	Unilever	Shareholder & Consultant	None	
Dr C Bartlett	None		None	
Dr Mary Cooke	None		None	
Professor C S F Easmon	None		None	
Dr P Fine	None		None	
Dr M Hinton	None		University of Bristol	Specific research projects undertaken by the University
Miss J Morris	None		None	
Mrs S Payne	None		None	
Mr E Ramsden	None		None	
Dr T Roberts	None		None	
Professor I M Smith	Duphor Veterinary Limited	Receives payment in cash for occasional work	None	
Mr M Verstringhe	Catering and Allied Services (International) Ltd.	Chairman	None	
	de Blank Restaurants	Director		
	Trustees Advanced Management Programme International	Chairman		
	European Catering Association International	President		
	Royal Society for the Encouragement of Arts, Manufacturers and Commerce.	Fellow		
	Quality Catering Partners - Zurich	Director		

23

REGISTER OF MEMBERS' INTERESTS

MEMBER	PERSONAL INTERESTS		NON-PERSONAL INTERESTS	
	Name of Company	Nature of Interest	Name of Company	Nature of Interest
HUMAN EPIDEMIOLOGY WORKING GROUP				
Dr B Bannister	None		None	
Dr J Cowden	Ladbroke Group plc	Shareholder	None	
	Reckitt and Colman plc	Shareholder		
	Sears plc	Shareholder		
	Thames Water plc	Shareholder		
	Young and Co's Brewery plc	Shareholder		
Prof R Feldman	None		None	
Mr W Reilly	Marks and Spencer plc	Shareholder	None	
Dr B Rowe	None		None	
FARM ANIMALS AND ABATTOIR SURVEILLANCE WORKING GROUP				
Dr T J Humphrey	None		None	
Dr A M Johnston	None		Food Safety Advisory Centre	Independent Advisory Panel Member
			Specific projects undertaken by the Royal Veterinary College	Independent advisor and liaison on behalf of the Royal Veterinary College
Dr D R Williams	None		None	

24

REGISTER OF MEMBERS' INTERESTS

MEMBER	PERSONAL INTERESTS		NON-PERSONAL INTERESTS	
	Name of Company	Nature of Interest	Name of Company	Nature of Interest
FOOD PROCESSING SURVEILLANCE WORKING GROUP				
Mr D Atherton	None		Princes Ltd	Representative on Campden FDRA and Leatherhead Food RA
Mr B M Bruce	Christian Salvesen plc	Shareholder	Christian Salvesen	Representative on various Trade Associations and Research Associations (UKAFFP, Campden FDRA and Leatherhead Food RA)
Mrs C Endacott-Pa mer	None		Representative on various Trade Associations and Research Associations (CFA, BMMA, CFDRA,and LFRA).	
Mr C Morrison	UB Ross Youngs	Shareholder	Representative on various Trade Associations	
Mrs L Pugh	None		Husbands business is "Quality Matters" a consultancy specialising in Food Quality Assurance for a variety of food companies.	
Mr D Smith	None		None	
RETAIL, CATERING AND CONSUMER SURVEILLANCE WORKING GROUP				
Dr L Ackerley	Hygiene Audit Systems Ltd. (Provides consultancy and training in the fields of health and safety and food safety.) The Public Health Company Ltd. (A consultancy providing environmental health services for local authorities and other public services.	Director and Shareholder	None	

25

REGISTER OF MEMBERS' INTERESTS

MEMBER	PERSONAL INTERESTS		NON-PERSONAL INTERESTS	
	Name of Company	Nature of Interest	Name of Company	Nature of Interest
Miss H Asmah	Tesco Stores Ltd	Shareholder	Tesco Stores Ltd	Tesco has a technical centre which can undertake commercial testing for external organisations.
Dr J Corry	J Sainsbury plc	Shareholder (Former employee)	University of Bristol	Specific research projects undertaken by the University
Mr W Davidson	Thames Water plc	Shareholder	None	
Dr J de Louvois	None		None	
Dr M Gasson	None		Institute of Food Research (IFR).	Specific research projects undertaken by IFR.
Mr T Miller	Whitbread plc	Shareholder. Owns shares in other firms, whose work does not impinge on the work of the Retail, Catering and Consumer Working Group.		
Mr M Norman	None		None	
Dr S Walker	None		None	

RESEARCH WORKING GROUP

MEMBER	PERSONAL INTERESTS		NON-PERSONAL INTERESTS	
Dr E O Caul	Dako Diagnostics	Consultant on clinical virology	None	

REGISTER OF MEMBERS' INTERESTS

MEMBER	PERSONAL INTERESTS		NON-PERSONAL INTERESTS	
	Name of Company	Nature of Interest	Name of Company	Nature of Interest
Dr I Farrell	None		None	
Dr M Stringer	None		A range of companies from the food and drink industry.	The structure of the Campden Food and Drink Research Association is such that a portion of the work is funded by the food and drink industries.
DOMESTIC PRACTICES SUB-GROUP				
Mrs W Browne	None		None	
Dr J Holland	None		None	
Mr M J Hudson	None		Centre for Appiled Microbiology and Research (CAMR)	Specific research projects undertaken by CAMR
Miss W L Spence	J Sainsbury plc	Shareholder	None	

Footnote: The declarations of personal interest shown in Appendix 2 are additional to those consequent on main employment which are shown in Appendix 1. The declarations of Working Group members who are shown in the full Steering Group are shown in the Steering Group section only. The declarations of Working Group members who are on the Domestic Sub-Group are shown under the respective Working Group.

SUMMARY OF ACTUAL EXPENDITURE ON SURVEILLANCE PROJECTS BY THE SGMSF WORKING GROUPS

Working Group	Project	Financial Year (rounded to the nearest £)					
		1990/91	1991/92	1992/93	1993/94	1994/95	TOTALS
HEWG	IID (PS)	£60,000	£10,000	NIL			£70,000
HEWG	IID Study in England	NA	NA	NA	£783,114	£910,913	£1,694,027
HEWG	Epidemiology of VTEC 0157 in the Sheffield area					£35,000	£35,000
RCCWG	Salad Bars (PS)	nil	£25,493	£33,794		£77,424	£136,711
RCCWG	Cream Cakes (PS)	nil	nil	£72,908			£72,908
RCCWG	Catering Premises (PS)	nil	nil	£3,940		£24,239	£28,179
RCCWG	Recovery of *Campylobacter* from surfaces (PS)	nil	nil	£4,375			£4,375
RCCWG	Survey of *Salmonella* in raw chicken on retail sale	NA	NA	NA	£69,780		£69,780
FPWG	Ready to Eat meat and meat products	nil	£3,628	£79,111	£59,908	£56,584	£199,231
FPWG	Canneries Study				£8,120	£56,400	£64,520
FPWG	Training of Samplers				£6,000	£13,855	£19,855
FPWG	MRM (PS)					£2,400	£2,400
FAAWG	Recovery of pathogens from animal carcases in abattoirs	nil	nil	£12,008	nil	£69,000	£81,008
FAAWG	*E.coli* in bovine faeces	nil	nil	nil	nil	£38,000	£38,000
Annual Totals		£60,000	£39,121	£206,136	£926,922	£1,273,815	£2,528,002

Grand Total for Whole Period £2,528,002

(PS) - Pilot Study

FOOD POISONING STATISTICS 1980-1994

Table 1: Food poisoning notifications Scotland, Northern Ireland and England and Wales 1980-94

Year	SCOTLAND			NORTHERN IRELAND			ENGLAND AND WALES				
	Mid-year pop.in 1,000s	Notifi-cations	+Rate	Mid-year pop.in 1,000s	Notifi-cations	+Rate	Mid-year pop.in 1,000s	Formal notifi-cations	+Rate	Formal notification + asc-ertained by other means	+Rate
1980	5,194	2299	44.3	1,533	114	7.4	49,603	10,318	20.8		
1981	5,180	2920	56.4	1,538	135	8.8	49,634	9,936	20.0		
1982	5,167	2880	55.7	1,538	198	12.9	49,613	9,964	20.1	14,253	28.7
1983	5,153	2632	51.1	1,543	128	8.3	49,681	12,273	24.7	17,735	35.7
1984	5,146	2391	46.5	1,550	144	9.3	49,810	13,247	26.6	20,702	41.6
1985	5,137	1967	38.3	1,558	158	10.1	49,990	13,143	26.3	19,242	38.5
1986	5,123	2436	47.6	1,567	273	17.4	50,162	16,502	32.9	23,948	47.7
1987	5,113	2480	48.5	1,575	423	26.9	50,321	20,363	40.5	29,331	58.3
1988	5,093	2998	58.9	1,578	302	19.1	50,487	27,826	55.1	39,713	78.7
1989	5,097	3197	62.7	1,583	501	31.6	50,678	38,086	75.2	52,557	103.7
1990	5,102	3024	59.3	1,589	819	51.5	50,869	36,945	72.6	52,145	102.5
1991	5,107	2938	57.5	1,601	636	39.7	51,100	35,291	69.1	52,543	102.8
1992	5,111	3317	64.9	1,618	915	56.6	51,277	42,551	83.0	63,347	123.5
1993	5,120	3255	63.6	1,632	954	58.5	51,439	44,271	86.1	68,587	133.3
1994	5,134*	4100*	79.9	1,628*	1,005*	61.7	51,612*	49,237*	95.4	82,587*	160.0

*Provisional figures

+Rate = per 100,000 population.

Population figures for 1980 are re-based estimates using the 1981 Census. Re-based estimates for 1981-1990, revised final estimates for 1991, and final estimates for 1992 and 1993 are based on the 1991 Census. Population figures for 1994 are 1992 projections.

Sources:
Population figures:-
Projections for England & Wales, Scotland and Northern Ireland - Government Actuary's Department.
Scotland Estimates - General Register Office for Scotland
Northern Ireland Estimates - General Register Office for Northern Ireland
England and Wales Estimates - Office of Population Censuses and Surveys
Food Poisoning Notifications:- OPCS, SCIEH and DHSS-NI

Table 2: *Campylobacter*: **Laboratory reports of faecal isolates 1981-1994**

Year	Scotland Reports to SCIEH		Northern Ireland Reports to DHSS (NI)		England & Wales Reports to CDSC	
	No.	rate/100,000 population	No.	rate/100,000 population	No.	rate/100,000 population
1981	1887	36.4	19	1.2	12168	24.5
1982	1922	37.2	24	1.6	12797	25.8
1983	1895	36.8	45	2.9	17278	34.8
1984	2181	42.4	58	3.7	21018	42.2
1985	2563	49.9	90	5.8	23572	47.2
1986	2372	46.3	73	4.7	24809	49.5
1987	2740	53.6	122	7.7	27310	54.3
1988	2906	57.1	173	11.0	28761	57.0
1989	3080	60.4	192	12.1	32526	64.2
1990	3625	71.1	244	15.4	34552	68.0
1991	3430	67.2	306	19.1	32636	63.9
1992	4915	96.2	419	25.9	38552	75.2
1993	4001	78.1	354	21.7	39383*	76.6
1994	4146	80.8	443*	27.2	44315*	85.9

Source: PHLS-CDSC, SCIEH and DHSS (NI)

* - Provisional figures

Table 3: *Salmonella*: Laboratory reports of faecal isolates 1981-1994

Year	All Salmonellas[1]		*S. typhimurium*		*S. enteritidis* (all phage types)		*S. enteritidis* PT4	
	No.	Rate/ 100,000 population	No.	Rate/ 100,000 population	No.	Rate/ 100,000 population	No.	Rate/ 100,000 population
A. Scotland Reports to SCIEH								
1981	2526	48.8	1117	21.6	250	4.8	37	0.7
1982	2621	50.7	1286	24.9	279	5.4	42	0.8
1983	2288	44.4	1201	23.3	319	6.2	80	1.6
1984	2221	43.2	1069	20.8	433	8.4	183	3.6
1985	1690	32.9	689	13.4	528	10.3	138	2.7
1986	2015	39.3	649	12.7	619	12.1	283	5.5
1987	2286	44.7	679	13.3	940	18.4	587	11.5
1988	2580	50.7	737	14.5	1345	26.4	910	17.9
1989	2578	50.6	552	10.8	1402	27.5	1116	21.9
1990	2441	47.8	606	11.9	1241	24.3	1083	21.2
1991	2330	45.6	503	9.8	1264	24.8	1101	21.6
1992	2992	58.5	662	13.0	1618	31.7	1309	25.6
1993	2919	57.0	527	10.3	1797	35.1	1512	29.5
1994	2973	57.9	610	11.9	1703	33.2	1364	26.6
B. Northern Ireland Reports to PHLS								
1981	69	4.5	39	2.5	7	0.5	3	0.2
1982	58	3.8	35	2.3	2	0.1	1	0.1
1983	87	5.6	50	3.2	12	0.8	4	0.3
1984	79	5.1	37	2.4	10	0.6	7	0.5
1985	85	5.5	49	3.1	13	0.8	9	0.6
1986	259	16.5	151	9.6	90	5.7	76	4.9
1987	422	26.8	150	9.5	235	14.9	207	13.1
1988	253	16.0	72	4.6	150	9.5	126	8.0
1989	190	12.0	40	2.5	96	6.1	82	5.2
1990	296	18.6	52	3.3	216	13.6	210	13.2
1991	160	10.0	39	2.4	89	5.6	69	4.3
1992	195	12.1	46	2.8	123	7.6	110	6.8
1993	174	10.7	34	2.1	125	7.7	101	6.2
1994	199	12.2	62	3.8	102	6.3	82	5.0
C. England and Wales Reports to PHLS								
1981	10251	20.7	3992	8.0	1087	2.2	395	0.8
1982	12322	24.8	6089	12.3	1101	2.2	413	0.8
1983	15155	30.5	7785	15.7	1774	3.6	823	1.7
1984	14727	29.6	7264	14.6	2071	4.2	1362	2.7
1985	13330	26.7	5478	11.0	3095	6.2	1771	3.5
1986	16976	33.8	7094	14.4	4771	9.5	2971	5.9
1987	20532	40.8	7660	15.2	6858	13.6	4962	9.9
1988	27478	54.4	6444	12.8	15427	30.6	12522	24.8
1989	29998	59.2	7306	14.4	15773	31.1	12931	25.5
1990	30112	59.2	5451	10.7	18840	37.0	16151	31.8
1991	27693	54.2	5331	10.4	17460	34.2	14693	28.8
1992	31355	61.1	5401	10.5	20094	39.2	16987	33.1
1993	30650	59.6	4778	9.3	20254	39.4	17258	33.6
1994	30428	59.0	5523	10.7	17370	33.7	13782	26.7

[1] - All Salmonellas excluding *S. typhi* and *S. paratyphi* - Scotland, Northern Ireland, England & Wales.

  1981-1988 LEP (formerly DEP) data as in Richmond Report Part 1 for England and Wales

  1988-1991 LEP (formerly DEP) data as in PHLS/SVS Update on *Salmonella* Infection, Editions 2,6,10

  1992-1994 PHLS *Salmonella* data set (1993 & 1994 data provisional)

SOURCE:PHLS,SCIEH

Table 4: Human listeriosis:- Scotland, Northern Ireland, England and Wales 1980-1994

Year	SCOTLAND No.	NORTHERN IRELAND No.	ENGLAND AND WALES No.
1980	12	N/A	75
1981	7	N/A	86
1982	10	2	75
1983	16	2	111
1984	10	1	112
1985	18	0	136
1986	10	2	129
1987	39	6	238
1988	40	11	278
1989	31	5	237
1990	15	3	116
1991	12	3	127
1992	15	2	106
1993	12	4	102
1994	12	1*	112*

Source: PHLS-CDSC, SCIEH.
N/A - not available
* - Provisional figures

Notes:

England, Wales and Northern Ireland
Prior to 1990 *Listeria* data was not computerised routinely, but recorded manually. In 1990 a computerised database was established using data ascertained via the national voluntary laboratory reporting scheme and information on isolates *L. monocytogenes* sent to the PHLS *Listeria* Reference Unit (LRU) for confirmation and typing.

During 1994 a reconciliation exercise of all data reported to the Communicable Disease Surveillance Centre (CDSC) and the *Listeria* Reference Unit between 1983 to the present was performed. During the course of this exercise duplicate reports were eliminated and there was mutual exchange of a handful of cases reported either to CDSC or LRU and not previously known to the other reporting scheme.

Scotland
Figures for Scotland represent all cases ascertained based on reports to the Scottish Centre for Infection and Environmental Health, cultures submitted to PHLS *Listeria* Reference Unit, and Hospital Deaths and Discharges recorded in the Scottish Morbidity Record schemes. This has resulted in some alterations in annual totals compared with those reported previously.

Table 5: *E. coli* 0157 Laboratory reports of faecal isolates 1982-1994

Year	SCOTLAND		NORTHERN IRELAND		ENGLAND & WALES	
	No.	rate/100,000 population	No.	rate/100,000 population	No.	rate/100,000 population
1982	N/A	N/A	N/A	N/A	1	<.01
1983	N/A	N/A	N/A	N/A	6	0.01
1984	3	0.06	N/A	N/A	9	0.02
1985	3	0.06	N/A	N/A	50	0.10
1986	4	0.08	N/A	N/A	76	0.15
1987	12	0.23	N/A	N/A	89	0.18
1988	39	0.77	0	0.00	49	0.10
1989	87	1.71	1	0.06	119	0.23
1990	173	3.39	1	0.06	250	0.49
1991	202	3.96	2	0.12	361	0.71
1992	115	2.25	1	0.06	470	0.92
1993	119	2.32	2	0.12	385	0.75
1994	242	4.71	3*	0.18	411*	0.80

Source: PHLS-LEP, SCIEH, DHSS (NI)
N/A - not available
* - Provisional figures

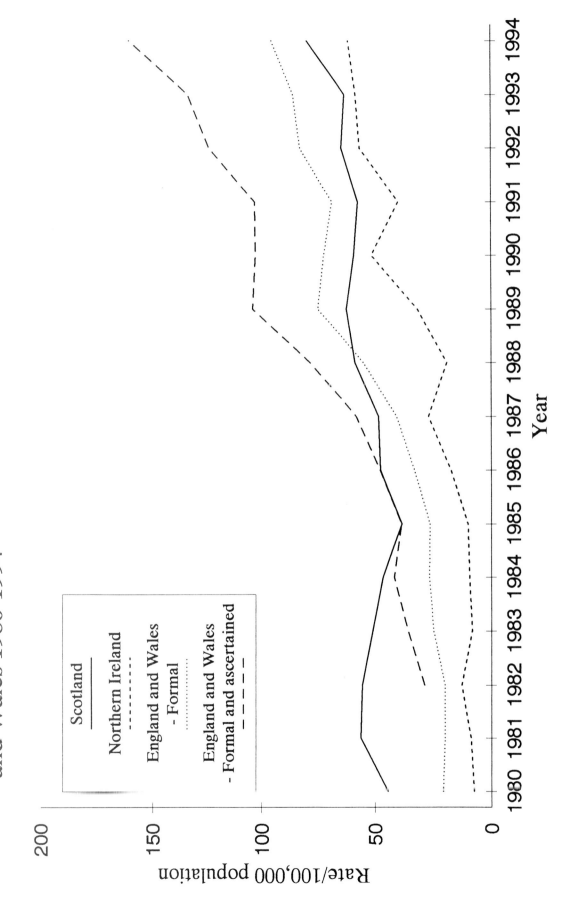

Figure 1: Food poisoning notifications: Scotland, Northern Ireland and England and Wales 1980-1994

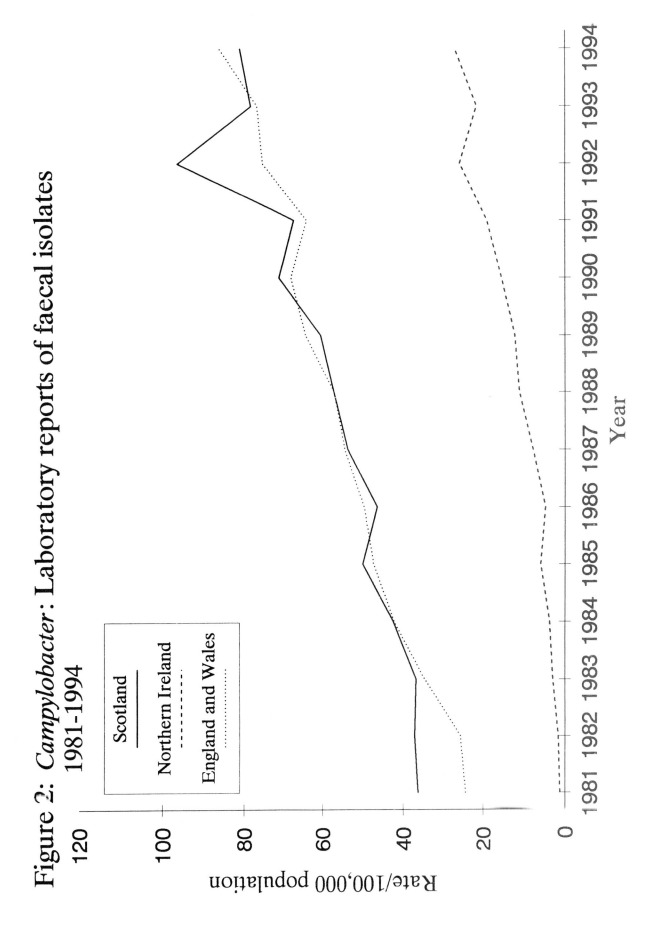

Figure 2: *Campylobacter*: Laboratory reports of faecal isolates 1981-1994

Scotland
Northern Ireland
England and Wales

Rate/100,000 population

120 100 80 60 40 20 0

1981 1982 1983 1984 1985 1986 1987 1988 1989 1990 1991 1992 1993 1994

Year

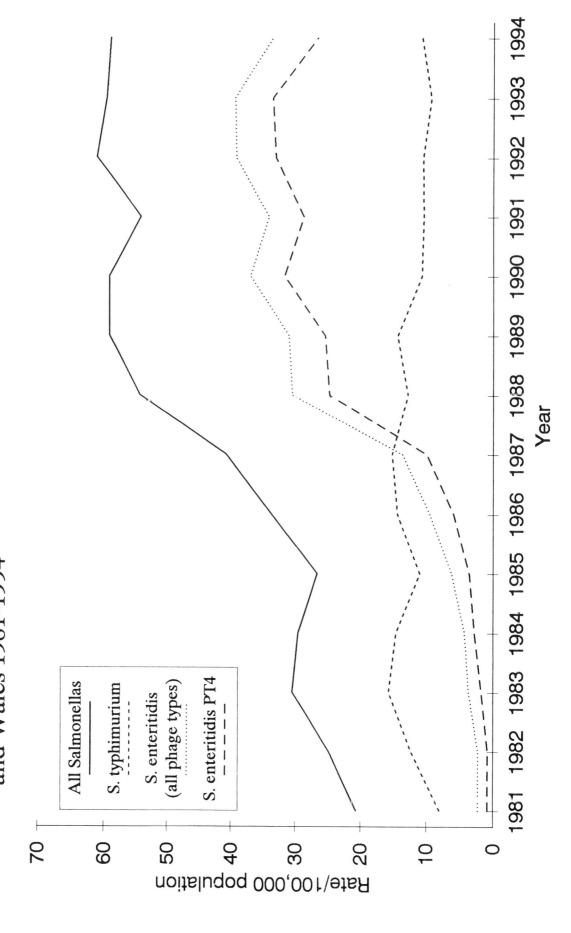

Figure 3: *Salmonella*: Laboratory reports of faecal isolates in England and Wales 1981-1994

Figure 4: *Salmonella*: Laboratory reports of faecal isolates in Scotland 1981-1994

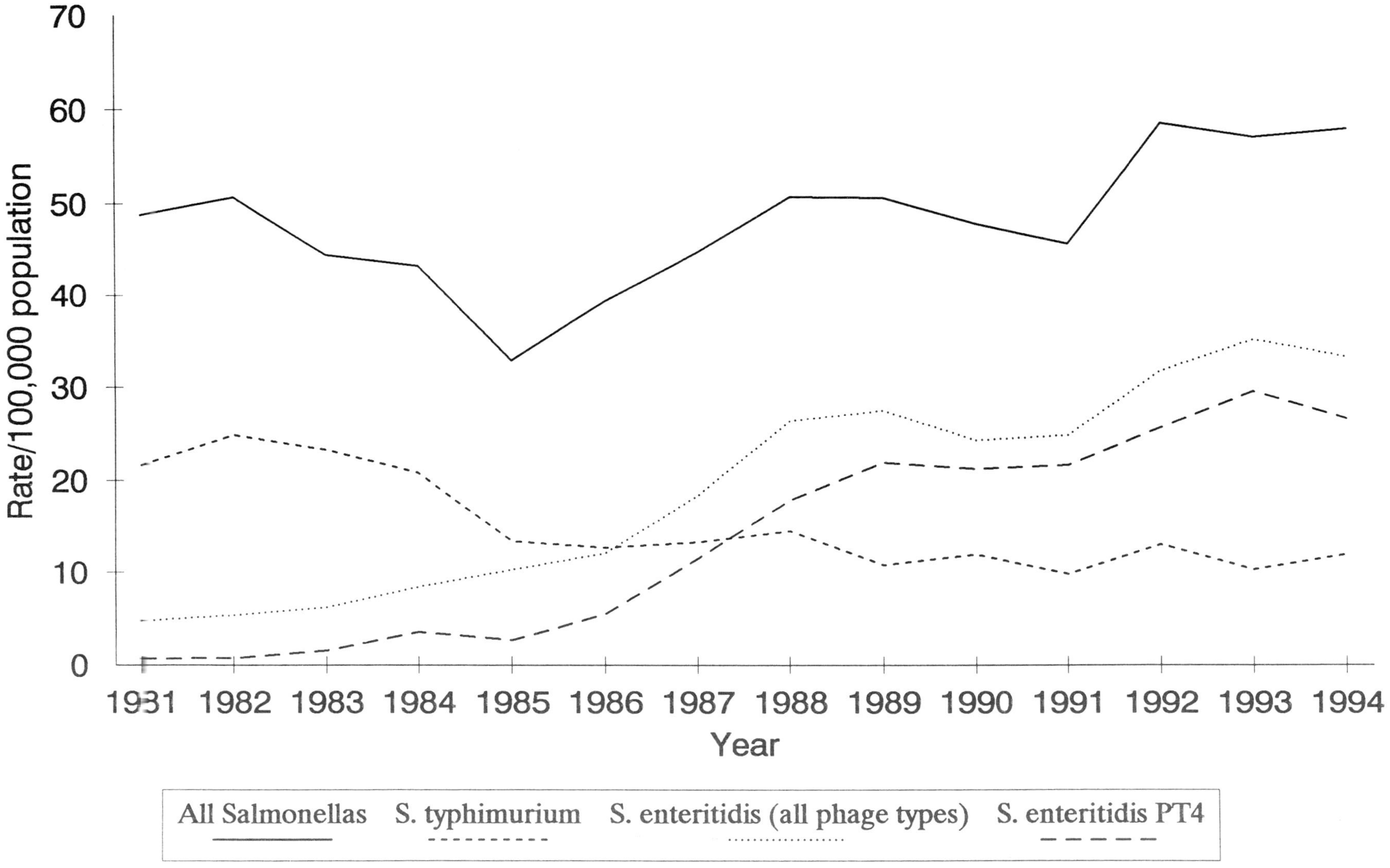

All Salmonellas   S. typhimurium   S. enteritidis (all phage types)   S. enteritidis PT4

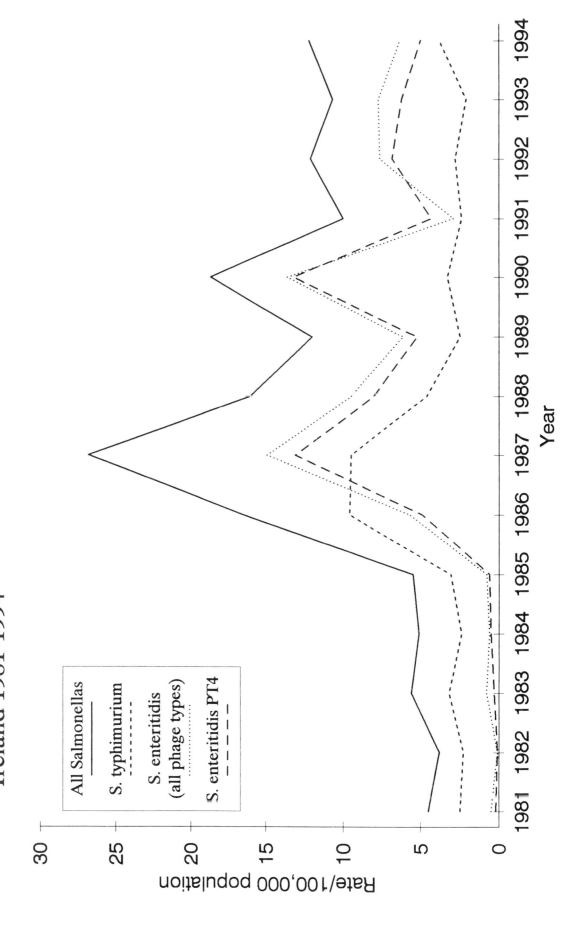

Figure 5: *Salmonella*: Laboratory reports of faecal isolates in Northern Ireland 1981-1994

| All Salmonellas |
| S. typhimurium |
| S. enteritidis (all phage types) |
| S. enteritidis PT4 |

Rate/100,000 population

Year

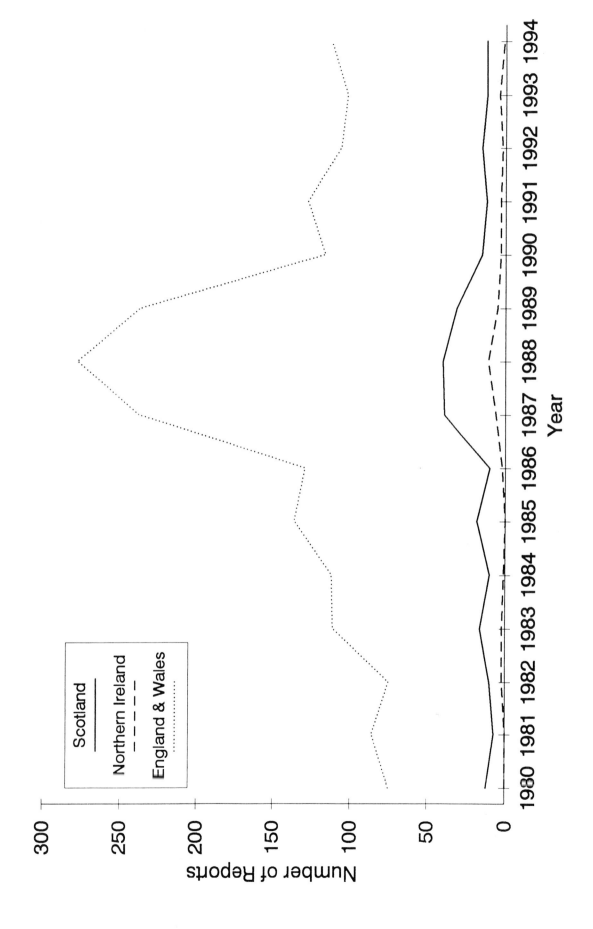

Figure 6: Human listeriosis: 1980-1994

Number of Reports

Year

Scotland
Northern Ireland
England & Wales

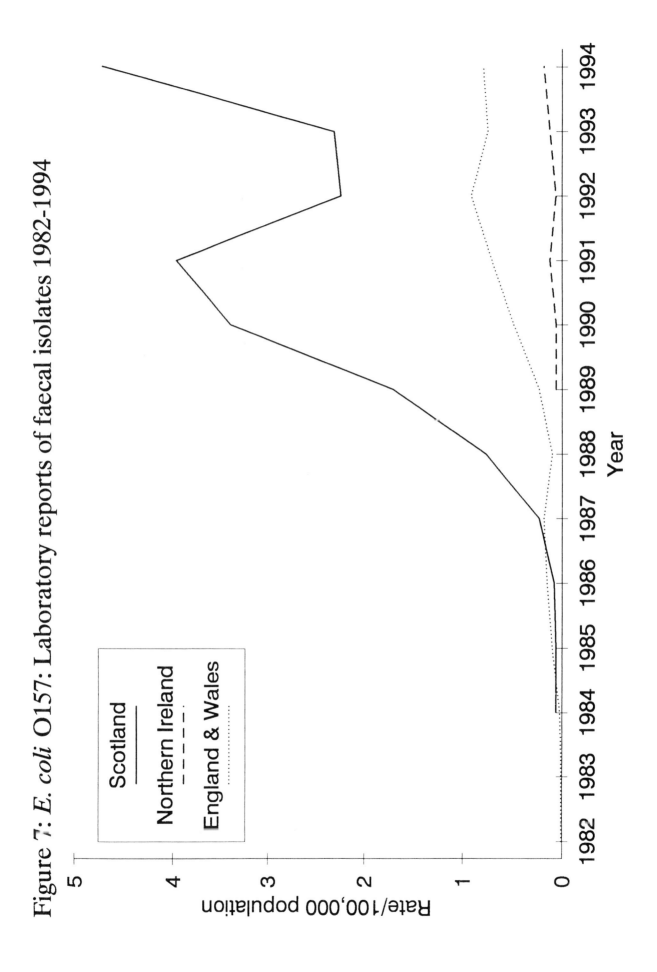

Figure 7: *E. coli* O157: Laboratory reports of faecal isolates 1982-1994

Scotland

Northern Ireland

England & Wales

Rate/100,000 population

Year

Table 1: Salmonellosis: Incidents of *Salmonella* in cattle in Great Britain and Northern Ireland 1980 - 1994

Year	All Salmonellas		*S. typhimurium*		*S. enteritidis*	
	GB	NI	GB	NI	GB	NI
1980	1374	37	708	8	5	0
1981	1484	49	845	15	9	0
1982	1618	74	877	29	11	0
1983	1962	76	1215	30	2	0
1984	1763	112	1174	25	3	1
1985	1871	133	1208	37	3	1
1986	1553	121	954	46	4	3
1987	1243	153	596	33	14	3
1988	1298	95	604	7	14	2
1989	1298	192	570	13	24	2
1990	1387	218	613	7	31	0
1991	1051	192	388	12	20	1
1992	940	174	342	16	13	0
1993	1442	74	677	7	21	0
1994*	1894	254	994	3	28	3

Source: MAFF in "*Salmonella* in Animal and Poultry Production" and DANI

* Provisional figures for 1994

In 1993 a new system for recording incidents was introduced. Data for 1993 and 1994 is not directly comparable with that for 1980-1992

An incident is defined as the reported isolation of *Salmonella* from an animal, group of animals or their environment under the Zoonoses Order 1975/1989 which can be related to identifiable animals. If more than one species is infected from a common source, separate incidents are recorded for each species. Many isolations from livestock are incidental too the investigation of other conditions or are reported as a result of routine monitoring of clinically healthy animals or poultry. The number of incidents therefore represent an unknown proportion of both clinical and subclinical infections occurring in the population at risk and may only be used to indicate trends.

Table 2: Salmonellosis: Incidents of *Salmonella* in sheep in Great Britain and Northern Ireland 1980 - 1994

Year	All Salmonellas		S. typhimurium		S. enteritidis	
	GB	NI	GB	NI	GB	NI
1980	78	2	1	1	2	0
1981	86	3	25	1	1	0
1982	193	19	58	11	3	0
1983	143	5	51	1	1	0
1984	149	5	51	1	1	0
1985	159	8	53	3	0	0
1986	153	15	48	7	3	2
1987	187	27	34	5	3	1
1988	189	9	29	1	7	0
1989	157	23	28	7	10	0
1990	194	19	38	2	7	0
1991	176	30	36	10	10	0
1992	106	15	23	2	1	0
1993	103	2	35	0	4	0
1994*	186	3	72	0	3	0

Source: MAFF in "*Salmonella* in Animal and Poultry Production" and DANI

* Provisional figures for 1994

In 1993 a new system for recording incidents was introduced. Data for 1993 and 1994 is not directly comparable with that for 1980-1992

Table 3: Salmonellosis: Incidents of *Salmonella* in pigs in Great Britain and Northern Ireland 1980 - 1994

Year	All Salmonellas		*S. typhimurium*		*S. enteritidis*	
	GB	NI	GB	NI	GB	NI
1980	143	30	32	3	1	1
1981	126	20	33	3	2	0
1982	159	15	39	5	1	0
1983	185	20	45	5	2	1
1984	167	20	50	3	0	0
1985	158	30	48	3	2	0
1986	159	27	55	4	2	3
1987	124	20	36	8	2	1
1988	100	14	34	4	1	0
1989	206	20	88	2	3	1
1990	228	20	87	0	5	0
1991	232	21	107	2	1	0
1992	261	25	149	2	8	0
1993	334	8	216	1	0	0
1994*	355	12	225	3	3	0

Source: MAFF in "*Salmonella* in Animal and Poultry Production" and DANI

* Provisional figures for 1994

In 1993 a new system for recording incidents was introduced. Data for 1993 and 1994 is not directly comparable with that for 1980-1992

Table 4: Salmonellosis: Incidents of *Salmonella* in domestic fowl in Great Britain and Northern Ireland 1980 - 1994

Year	All Salmonellas		S. typhimurium		S. enteritidis	
	GB	NI	GB	NI	GB	NI
1980	1433	66	176	15	7	0
1981	732	73	77	10	8	0
1982	616	76	58	18	8	0
1983	514	65	92	6	1	1
1984	446	64	135	12	0	0
1985	456	93	96	27	15	0
1986	519	177	130	66	36	50
1987	497	110	92	31	111	45
1988	838	54	78	10	401	9
1989	1530	56	131	6	738	7
1990	1906	55	107	6	843	6
1991	1803	97	112	12	816	3
1992	1447	97	103	17	683	2

Year	All Salmonellas		S. typhimurium		S. enteritidis	
1993	1068	59	30	15	492	4
1994*	715	N/A	30	N/A	214	N/A

Source: MAFF in "*Salmonella* in Animal and Poultry Production" and DANI

* Provisional figures for 1994

In 1993 a new system for recording incidents was introduced. Data for 1993 and 1994 is not directly comparable with that for 1980 - 1992

Table 5: Salmonellosis: Incidents of *Salmonella* in all poultry in Great Britain 1993 and 1994

Type of poultry	1993			1994*		
	All Sal.	St	Se	All Sal.	St	Se
Broilers	590	17	303	396	14	124
Broiler Breeder	381	8	164	227	10	76
Layer Breeder	47	5	16	10	2	3
Layers	43	0	8	51	0	1
Unknown Fowl Type	7	0	1	31	4	10
Turkeys	377	9	1	401	11	65
Ducks	328	87	88	123	33	30
Geese	5	0	1	4	2	1
Other Birds	172	96	7	190	79	18
Total	**1950**	**222**	**589**	**1433**	**155**	**328**

All Sal. = All *Salmonella* serotypes   Se = *S. enteritidis*   St = *S. typhimurium*

Source: MAFF

* Provisional figures for 1994

Table 6: Incidents of *Salmonella typhimurium* DT104 reported from cattle in
Great Britain, 1985 - 1994

Year	All Salmonellas	*S. typhimurium*	*S. typhimurium* DT 104
1985	1871	1208	15
1986	1553	954	11
1987	1243	596	27
1988	1298	604	32
1989	1298	570	47
1990	1387	613	28
1991	1051	388	109
1992	940	342	174
1993	1442	677	306
1994*	1894	994	587

Source: MAFF

* Provisional figures for 1994

Table 7: Incidents of *Salmonella typhimurium* DT104 reported from sheep in
Great Britain, 1985 - 1994

Year	All Salmonellas	*S. typhimurium*	*S. typhimurium* DT 104
1985	159	53	0
1986	153	48	1
1987	187	34	3
1988	189	29	1
1989	157	28	3
1990	194	38	2
1991	176	36	4
1992	106	23	4
1993	103	35	15
1994*	186	72	46

Source: MAFF

* Provisional figures for 1994

Table 8: Incidents of *Salmonella typhimurium* DT104 reported from pigs in Great Britain, 1985 - 1994

Year	All Salmonellas	*S. typhimurium*	*S. typhimurium* DT 104
1985	158	48	1
1986	159	55	1
1987	124	36	0
1988	100	34	0
1989	206	88	0
1990	228	87	0
1991	232	107	4
1992	261	149	14
1993	334	216	26
1994*	355	225	62

Source: MAFF

* Provisional figures for 1994

Table 9: Incidents of *Salmonella typhimurium* DT104 reported from poultry in Great Britain, 1993-1994

	1993				1994*			
	All Salmonella	ST	ST DT104	SE	All Salmonella	ST	ST DT104	SE
Broilers	590	17	6	303	396	14	14	124
Broiler Breeders	381	8	0	164	227	10	2	76
Layer	47	5	2	16	10	2	0	3
Layer Breeder	43	0	0	8	51	0	0	1
Fowl Unknown Type	7	0	0	1	31	4	2	10
Turkeys	377	9	2	1	401	11	6	65
Ducks	328	87	0	88	123	33	4	30
Geese Bird	5	0	0	1	4	2	2	1
Other Bird Type	172	96	0	7	190	79	2	18
TOTAL	**1950**	**222**	**10**	**589**	**1433**	**155**	**34**	**328**

All Salmonella	= All *Salmonella* serotypes
ST	= *Salmonella typhimurium*
ST DT104	= *Salmonella typhimurium* DT104
SE	= *Salmonella enteritidis*

Source: MAFF

* Provisional figures 1994

Table 10: The overall *Salmonella* contamination rates found in various types of feedingstuffs and raw ingredients in Great Britain during 1993 and 1994

Animal feedingstuffs of raw ingredient	No of tests carried out		No of tests positive		Percentage tests positive	
	1993	1994*	1993	1994*	1993	1994*
Processed animal protein sampled at a protein processor in GB.	4,855	10,203	108	220	2.2%	2.2%
GB and imported Processed animal protein sampled at feed compounders.	6,316	6,137	172	254	2.7%	4.7%
Linseed meal, rapeseed meal, soyabean meal and sunflower meal sampled at GB crushing premises.	3,708	2,709	145	127	3.9%	4.7%
Oilseed meals and products sampled at feedmills for incorporation into animal feedingstuffs.	13,600	12,460	1,072	616	7.9%	4.9%
Non-oilseed meal vegetable products.	11,601	14,422	248	289	2.1%	2.0%
Ruminant compound feed.	3,379	3,235	159	111	4.7%	3.4%
Pig compound feed.	5,617	6,598	118	239	2.1%	3.6%
Poultry compound feed.	9,972	14,256	268	389	2.7%	2.7%
Protein concentrate.	1,301	1,724	41	64	3.2%	3.7%
Minerals/other	1,222	949	5	5	0.4%	0.5%

Source: MAFF

* Provisional figures for 1994

Table 11: The number of isolates of *Salmonella enteritidis* and *Salmonella typhimurium* reported from animal feedingstuffs in Great Britain, 1991 - 1994

Type of material	1991		1992		1993		1994*	
	Se	St	Se	St	Se	St	Se	St
Finished feed	0	15	6	15	5	9	4	25
Animal protein	24	0	0	0	0	1	0	4
Vegetable protein	4	2	2	8	7	15	1	6
Minerals	0	0	0	0	0	0	0	0
Miscellaneous	0	0	2	5	2	1	0	4
TOTAL	28	7	10	28	14	26	5	39

Se = *Salmonella enteritidis*   St = *Salmonella typhimurium*

Source: MAFF

* Provisional figures 1994

Table 12: Results of MAFF testing of home produced processed animal protein in Great Britain under the Processed Animal Protein Order 1989

	1988	1989	1990	1991	1992	1993	1994*
No of samples tested	847	1,674	1,388	1,360	1,318	1,274	1,066
No positive all serotypes	44	88	40	46	22	26	27
No of S.enteritidis	1	8	1	2	3	1	0
No of S.typhimurium	5	4	0	0	0	0	0
% of samples positive	5.2	5.3	2.9	3.3	1.7	2.0	2.5

Source: MAFF

* Provisional figures for 1994

Table 13: Incidents of listeriosis in animals diagnosed by VI Centres in Great Britain and Northern Ireland 1980 - 1994

Year	Cattle		Sheep		Pigs		Birds		Misc.		All species	
	GB	NI	GB	NI	GB	NI	GB	NI	GB	NI	GB	NI
1980	27	NR	78	NR	2	NR	5	NR	3	NR	115	NR
1981	22	NR	73	NR	3	NR	2	NR	6	NR	106	NR
1982	53	NR	161	NR	1	NR	4	NR	9	NR	228	NR
1983	42	NR	196	NR	2	NR	2	NR	21	NR	263	NR
1984	41	NR	217	NR	1	NR	1	NR	15	NR	275	NR
1985	24	NR	272	NR	3	NR	1	NR	12	NR	312	NR
1986	50	NR	406	NR	4	NR	6	NR	19	NR	485	NR
1987	49	NR	351	NR	2	NR	2	NR	27	NR	431	NR
1988	50	NR	347	NR	1	NR	6	NR	22	NR	426	NR
1989	73	NR	359	NR	0	NR	7	NR	34	NR	473	NR
1990	57	NR	212	NR	0	NR	1	NR	15	NR	286	NR
1991	46	NR	245	NR	2	NR	2	NR	15	NR	310	NR
1992	41	NR	190	NR	3	NR	9	NR	25	NR	268	NR
1993	27	10	159	10	0	0	3	0	9	0	198	NR
1994*	21	4	194	15		0	3	1	11	1	229	21

Source: MAFF, WOAD, SOAFD in "Veterinary Investigation Diagnosis Analysis" (VIDA) and DANI

* Provisional figures
NR = Not recorded

Table 14: Incidents of Cryptosporidiosis in animals diagnosed by VI Centres in Great Britain and Northern Ireland 1980 - 1994

Year		Great Britain				Northern Ireland		
		Cattle	Sheep	All		Cattle	Sheep	All
1980		NR	NR	NR		NR	NR	NR
1981		NR	NR	NR		NR	NR	NR
1982		NR	NR	NR		NR	NR	NR
1983		NR	NR	NR		NR	NR	NR
1984		256	26	282		NR	NR	NR
1985		448	51	499		NR	NR	NR
1986		438	57	495		NR	NR	NR
1987		795	88	883		NR	NR	NR
1988		853	162	1015		NR	NR	NR
1989		916	156	1072		34	8	42
1990		852	102	954		47	7	54
1991		912	106	1018		64	14	78
1992		1171	94	1265		61	16	77
1993		1543	101	1554		84	7	91
1994*		1602	154	1756		170	10	180

Source: MAFF, WOAD, SOAFD in "Veterinary Investigation Diagnosis Analysis" (VIDA) and DANI

* Provisional figures
NR = Not recorded

STEERING GROUP ON THE MICROBIOLOGICAL SAFETY OF FOOD (SGMSF)

GUIDELINES ON STUDY PROTOCOLS

<u>Introduction</u>

1.   This document gives guidance on the content and format of surveillance study protocols. It is designed to assist the SGMSF Working Groups in developing study protocols that contain the information identified by the Research Working Group (RWG) as essential. It also encourages the use of standardised approaches to microbiological surveillance, where appropriate. **Surveillance** in the SGMSF context refers to the gathering and interpretation of information relevant to the microbiological safety of food. It may include investigation of specific foods or food ingredients, pathogens, processes, practices or associated perceptions and behaviour. Such surveillance will usually be carried out on a non-routine basis, but as the SGMSF's surveillance programme develops, some studies may be repeated to assist in the identification of trends.

2.   The guidance should be read in conjunction with *Methods for Use in Microbiological Surveillance* published by the SGMSF on 16 June 1994.

<u>Scope of Guidance</u>

3.   The guidance is split into seven sections:

-     types of surveillance studies;

-     essential elements of a protocol;

-     statistics;

-     sampling methods, including chilling;

-     microbiological methods, including a recommended core list of pathogens to be looked for in studies;

-     laboratory accreditation and proficiency schemes; and

-     archiving of samples, isolates and associated information.

<u>Types of Surveillance Studies</u>

4.   The SGMSF has identified four types of surveillance studies and agreed the following definitions for them:

(a). <u>Pilot Study</u>: a study designed to assess the feasibility of a proposed surveillance project and assist with its design. A pilot study would be used to identify and/or test solutions to problems in some or all of the elements of a project protocol, including training and supervision of samplers, sample collection, transport and storage, methods of analysis, and data handling and analysis. Such a study would **not** be designed to provide statistically reliable surveillance data and scientific inferences would not normally be drawn from pilot study results by the SGMSF or its Working Groups.

(h)   <u>Targeting Study</u>: a short-term surveillance exercise which could be used to test hypotheses on potential areas or topics of concern. Such studies would usually be too small in scale to produce statistically-valid data, so reassurance should not be implied from negative results. However, positive results might provide an indication of a potential microbiological problem and therefore the need for a larger scale survey.

(c). <u>Major Study</u>: a project intended to provide sufficient information to enable the SGMSF to make an assessment of the microbiological situation. Such a study would usually be conducted on a regional basis or would target specific aspects or sectors of the food group under scrutiny. Depending on the statistical validity of the data, study results might be judged by the Steering Group to be representative of the national situation.

(d). National Study: a project designed from the outset to provide scientifically valid data from which inferences can be drawn about the national situation.

Essential Elements of a Study Protocol

5.   A study protocol should contain the following essential elements:

(a).   an abstract of the project;

(b).   an explanation of the project's objectives;

(c).   a brief summary of any relevant literature;

(d).   a statistical explanation of the sampling size in relation to the project's objectives and the analyses of results to be done;

(e).   timescale of project, including key milestones;

(f).   sampling methodologies;

(g).   details of transportation of samples;

(h).   methods for microbiological analysis;

(i).   estimated costs of project;

(j).   plans for disclosure of results (including where these are adverse);

(k).   plans for training of samplers/laboratories;

(l).   guidance notes for samplers and laboratories, including questionnaires, checklists and other documentation;

(m).   plans for archiving of isolates and/or clinical samples; and.

(n).   legal aspects ie. the effect of any relevant legislation eg. the Zoonoses Order for isolations of *Salmonella*.

6.   When a protocol is submitted to the RWG for comment, the RWG has decided that it would be helpful if the Working Groups sent a microbiologist or other suitably qualified person to RWG meetings to assist discussion and answer any queries. Typically, this could be the Scientific Secretary of the Working Group, Working Group member(s) or proposed study contractors. For example, in the case of the Human Epidemiology Working Group (HEWG), this may be an epidemiologist; for all of the Working Groups' protocols, a statistician may sometimes need to be present.

Statistics

7.   The RWG held a statistics workshop in 1992 and issued guidance approved by the SGMSF to the other Working Groups. This is reproduced at **Annex 1**. It has been updated to take account of the SGMSF terminology for surveillance studies in paragraph 4 above. Additional guidance on calculating the weighted mean in the enumeration of micro-organisms is included in *Methods for Use in Microbiological Surveillance* (see paragraph 2 above).

8.   It is essential that Working Groups develop clear objectives for a study and obtain expert statistical and, where necessary, epidemiological advice at an early stage, if a statistically valid sampling frame is to be achieved. The protocol should contain an explanation of the statistical sampling frame in relation to the study's objectives.

9.   The SGMSF's policy is that 95% confidence intervals should normally be used. There may be cases where a lack of information about the product/process/premises/pathogens to be investigated make it impossible to calculate 95%

confidence intervals. In these cases, subject to statistical advice, smaller samples might be taken.

Sampling Methods

10. In the study protocol, there should be detailed information about sampling methods such as site, product, equipment, procedure, timing, storage and transportation. An example of sampling methods approved by the RWG is that used for a Retail, Catering and Consumer Surveillance Working Group study of potential contamination sites in catering premises (see **Annex 2**). The compendium of microbiological methods referred to in paragraph 2 above will be expanded in due course to include sampling methods endorsed by the RWG and SGMSF for use by the Working Groups.

11. Where validated sampling methods are available, these should be used and should include full references to the literature. The ICMSF publication, *"Microorganisms in Foods 2. Sampling for Microbiological Analysis: Principles and Specific Applications"* (Chapter 9, pages 114-123, 1986, 2nd ed. University of Toronto Press, Toronto, ISBN 0-8020-5693-8) is a useful source of reference for sampling techniques.

Core Group of Samplers

12. The Food Processing Surveillance Working Group (FPSWG) is recruiting a core group of approximately 100-150 samplers from Environmental Health Departments in England and Wales via Food Sampling Liaison Groups to be used in the national ready to eat meat and meat products study. The intention is that the core group of samplers may be available for use by the other Working Groups. The RWG will provide details of the core group of samplers to the other Working Groups when available.

Chilling of samples

13. The RWG recommends that, where necessary, chilling rather than freezing should be used for transportation and storage of samples before analysis. This is likely to have the least adverse effect on the viability of micro-organisms. Samples should be <u>transported and stored at temperatures not exceeding 4°C.</u> For transporting samples, samplers should use a coolbox capable of maintaining samples at temperatures not exceeding 4°C.

14. Laboratory refrigerators should have the capacity of maintaining the samples at the required temperature. The temperature of the chilled samples should be recorded on receipt at the laboratory and monitored at regular intervals during the storage period until microbiological examination is carried out.

15. Any deviation from the required temperature should be recorded and reported by the laboratory to the project team.

Microbiological Methods

16. The SGMSF has agreed that microbiological methods used should be :

- a national or international reference method;

- method otherwise validated by collaborative trial; or

- demonstrated by documented evidence to be equivalent or superior to the reference methods.

Methods for Use in Microbiological Surveillance

17. The SGMSF has published a compendium of microbiological methods entitled *Methods for Use in Microbiological Surveillance* (see paragraph 2 above). This compendium will be updated as necessary when additional methods are endorsed or currently endorsed methods are superseded. Working Groups should refer to the compendium when developing protocols to see if a suitable method has already been endorsed by the RWG and SGMSF. When it is proposed to use a method not already endorsed by the RWG and SGMSF, the method should be fully documented and in the format

used in the compendium, including the Vancouver system of citing references.

<u>Novel, Non-standard Methods</u>

18.   For novel, non-standard methods which are required to be used by a particular laboratory in Steering Group surveillance protocols, an inter-laboratory collaborative trial of the method and/or of the proficiency of the laboratory in the use of the method may be required. This will be assessed by the RWG on a case-by-case basis. In some situations this could provide data for the method to become validated. The RWG also recommend that, where appropriate, when non-standard methods are part of a protocol, specific guidance and training should be given to participating laboratories.

<u>Core List of Pathogens</u>

19.   The RWG recommends that, because of their association with human foodborne illness, the core list of pathogens for SGMSF surveillance studies is currently as follows:

- *Salmonella*;

- *Campylobacter*;

- *Escherichia coli* O157; and

- *Listeria monocytogenes.*

20.   There may be studies in which, for various reasons, Working Groups decide not to look for one or more of these pathogens. In these cases, the protocol should contain full and, if appropriate, referenced explanation for their omission.

<u>Sub-typing of Isolates</u>

21.   The SGMSF has agreed that all isolates should be sub-typed for epidemiological purposes. Specific reference to sub-typing should be made in study protocols. If necessary specialist reference laboratories should be used. (See also paragraph 27.7 in relation to the archiving of isolates of microorganisms).

Laboratory Accreditation and Proficiency Schemes

22.   The SGMSF has agreed that in order to ensure the quality of microbiological results obtained through the surveillance programme, participating laboratories should be NAMAS (National Measurement Accreditation Service) accredited for appropriate measurements. Where a participating laboratory is not NAMAS accredited, it should be accredited under another scheme of an acceptable standard. With regard to pathology laboratories examining clinical samples, the RWG considers the scheme run by CPA (UK) Ltd. accreditation, which requires participation in NEQAS, to be acceptable.

23.   The SGMSF does recognise the practical limitation of its recommendation above, and as an interim measure, recommends that laboratories:

23.1   demonstrate a commitment to acquiring accreditation within a realistic timescale. Such commitment would be judged by factors such as the quality systems already in place e.g. the quality manual, documentation of microbiological methods and the existence of a documented training scheme. The progress of the laboratory's application for accreditation would also be taken into consideration;

23.2   demonstrate successful participation in an appropriate external quality assessment scheme, such as one which is on the NAMAS Register of UK Proficiency Testing Schemes (chemistry/microbiology), to indicate their general standard of performance. NAMAS strongly encourage accredited laboratories to participate in an external quality assessment scheme. Details of NAMAS accredited food microbiology laboratories and the test methods covered by the accreditation are available in their Directory D3.

24. The SGMSF has considered the need at this stage for custom-designed EQA schemes using Steering Group methods, but it feels that this is not essential as existing schemes give sufficient assurance of the general proficiency of a laboratory. The Working Groups should, however, reserve the right to distribute customised samples for proficiency

testing using a specific method if this is judged necessary.

Approaches to NAMAS

25.   Approaches to NAMAS in relation to the SGMSF's surveillance programme should be channelled through the RWG. This should ensure consistency, and avoid duplication and confusion.

Archiving of Samples, Isolates and Associated Information

26.   The SGMSF has agreed that the archiving of clinical samples, isolates and associated information should be considered when a study is carried out, (eg. the study of infectious intestinal disease in England (IID)), as they will provide valuable and unique reference material for the future. Plans for archiving should be referred to in study protocols.

27.   The SGMSF has endorsed the following RWG recommendations in relation to archiving:

Samples

27.1 The need for archiving samples should be considered at the outset of the project. Where there are only limited quantities of samples which the Steering Group and funding department may wish to use in further studies, access to the central archive by outside bodies should be restricted as considered necessary by the Steering Group and funding department. Both these considerations can be assessed on a case-by-case basis. In general, the benefit of retaining original food or environmental samples, unlike clinical samples, is considered to be outweighed by the disadvantages.

27.2 The preservation techniques for faecal samples in the IID Study are defined in the IID microbiological protocol, an extract from which is attached at Annex C for reference.

Isolates of microorganisms

27.3 Isolates of all putative pathogens sought should be archived. Freezing at -70°C or colder with a cryopreservative is recommended as the technique of choice for maintaining the stability and viability of archived cultures and for preserving their genetic material.

27.4 Isolates from the IID study are being stored at -70°C with a cryopreservative as described in the IID study microbiological protocol. An extract from that protocol is attached at Annex C for reference.

27.5 Access by outside bodies to the central archive should generally be allowed only after publication of the final report of the study by the Steering Group.

27.6 There are likely to be cost advantages of scale which may be gained by centralising the archiving arrangement, as well as the benefit of unifying the collection of surveillance isolates. The RWG has therefore recommended that the Steering Group sets up a centralised archiving arrangement.

27.7 The Steering Group policy that isolates of putative pathogens should be sub-typed for epidemiological purposes, and that protocols should make specific provision for this, is still appropriate. However, whether this is necessary, or indeed possible, prior to archiving should be assessed on a case-by-case basis. The RWG is well placed to ensure a consistent approach as the surveillance programme progresses.

27.8 It is likely that participating microbiological laboratories may wish to retain their own local cultures of isolates sent to the central archive. There is no obvious reason for the Steering Group or the funding body to object to this and it would be very difficult to prevent it in any case. Publication of any work using these cultures should not precede the Steering Group's report, and the authors should be requested to make suitable acknowledgment of the Steering Group. Nevertheless, the Steering Group and the funding department may wish to consider, on a case-by-case basis, requests for early publication of results that are of sufficient interest or importance to justify this course of action.

Paper records

27.9 Hard copies of protocols, reports and contracts should be retained by funding bodies according to departmental policy. Reports of projects should be published so as to generate an ISBN and thereby involve the British Library facility.

Electronic data

27.10   Electronic copies of protocols, the full dataset and the report should be deposited at the Economic and Social Research Council Data Archive (ESRC) at Essex University which provides specialist electronic data archive facilities. The ESRC archive is able to maintain the data in a currently machine readable form and to make them available on-line to bona fide researchers on request. The timing of deposition of data should follow publication of the final report of the study by the Steering Group. Staff at the ESRC data archive should be consulted at an early stage for advice on necessary documentation etc. The ESRC publication *Preparing Data for Deposit with the ESRC Data Archive* provides useful guidance.

27.11   The archived dataset should not include personal details of individuals, e.g. names or addresses, or identifiable details of commercial organisations.

Cost and logistic implications

27.12   The cost and logistic implications of archiving should be considered by relevant Working Groups when developing protocols for surveillance projects. Any consequent decision about charging for access to archived samples or isolates should be taken by the funding department on a case-by-case basis.

RESEARCH WORKING GROUP

STATISTICAL GUIDANCE FOR MICROBIOLOGICAL SURVEILLANCE

Note: This guidance should be read in conjunction with paragraphs 4,7,8 and 9 of the main text.

SUMMARY

When conducting microbiological surveillance:

-   employ **Expert survey practitioners** and/or **statisticians;**

-   carry out a **"Brainstorming Session"** to explore objectives, requirements, causative factors and measurable effects;

-   establish clear but detailed **Objectives;**

-   identify **Target Population, Scope, Coverage, Effects to be measured or assessed, Required Resolution, controlled (risk) factors, measurable uncontrolled (risk) factors;**

-   choose or **pilot a sampling strategy,** probably with some combination of **cluster** and **stratified** sampling;

-   use **Pilot Studies** to clarify methods, feasibility, target population, standard deviation;

-   identify one or more **sampling frames;**

-   use **95% Confidence Intervals** for normal levels of assurance;

-   aim for **5% Level of Statistical Significance** for comparisons and hypothesis testing for normal levels of assurance;

-   use Confidence Intervals rather than Statistical Significance if there is a choice;

-   decide on **sample sizes** depending on **variability, resolution v confidence levels, hypothetical causative factors to be assessed;**

-   consider whether to use sophisticated **experimental designs.**

GUIDELINES

1.   A clear detailed set of objectives needs to be evolved for each study. Normally they should embrace the overall objectives of the surveillance programme with elaboration where necessary. However pilot or targeting studies would not cover as many objectives as a major or national study as they would only aim to answer some of the questions at issue.

2.   On the other hand, a Pilot Study should include objectives concerning such areas as methodology and feasibility which are certainly **not** part of the aims of the main study; indeed they are intended to resolve problems over its design and planning. For example, the objectives of the "Pilot Investigation of Infectious Intestinal Disease in the Population" include assessment of the feasibility of methods of patient recruitment.

3.   The Study Team should identify explicitly within the objectives or elsewhere:

   the **target population** - what animals, products, people ...

   the **scope** of the study and population - all of UK, including imports, only rural areas, over a short or extended time period? ...

   the **coverage** of the population - all or selected local authorities?, all slaughterhouses or a sample?

   what **measured effects** on the population are to be evaluated - concentrations of microorganisms, prevalence or relative risk of food poisoning ...

   the **resolution or resolving power or degree of discrimination** required for each of the measured effects? - eg maximum desired width of confidence interval for a concentration, minimum detectable difference in relative risks;

   the **controlled (risk) factors** (ie deliberately selected in the sampling scheme) which might affect results - region, "type" of processor, season, position in display cabinet, social class, sex ...

   other **measured, uncontrolled or wild-card (risk) factors** (ie observed but not deliberately selected in the sampling scheme) which could confound the results - laboratory, analytical method, kitchen hygiene ...

4.   It is recommended that the Project Board or Study Team charged with the execution of the study should consult statisticians or market research professionals with good acknowledged experience in designing, conducting and analysing surveys. The Team must choose a strategy for sampling the target population in compliance with the objectives such as those suggested above; they are likely to consider various schemes for **two-stage** sampling, with a mixture of **cluster** sampling of the **primary** units and **stratified** sampling within the clusters. In any case **a sampling frame** needs to be established. If necessary some sectors of the population should be over-represented to provide sufficient **resolving** power.

5.   The Study Team should consider whether to attempt some form of efficient and cost-saving but complex factorial **experimental design** or rely on a simpler but more expensive study.

6.   Such details are at the discretion of the Study Team. It is suggested that they arrange a **"brainstorming"** session to reveal factors and objectives; either in that or other meetings, they must cover all the issues considered in the previous few paragraphs.

A possible structure of the session is:

   1.   **Assemble ideas on objectives**
   2.   **Discuss and prioritise them**
   3.   **Identify a candidate list of cause/risk factors**

    4.   **Reduce list of factors to manageable size**

    5.   **Plan Pilot Trials**

7.   For most, if not all, surveys in the programme it will be necessary to perform pilot studies in order to produce a statistically valid sampling plan for larger studies. However, in some cases it may be possible to omit such studies if sufficient microbiological data is already available eg in the scientific literature, from previous surveillance studies etc.

Confidence Intervals - Normal Level to be 95%

8.   In general reported results of surveys should include the estimated **95% (two-sided) confidence interval** (bounded by **lower** and **upper 97.5%** confidence **limits**) associated with any estimated value such as concentration, rate of incidence, relative risk.

9.   The method used to determine a confidence interval should be appropriate and conform to accepted statistical practice. It is not always correct to use

value + or - 2 x standard-deviation, especially for low rates of incidence or for relative risk. **One-sided** bounds (eg Upper confidence limit, UCL) should be at a level of **97.5%.**

10.   It is always **acceptable** to use the more stringent level of 99% as the 95% Confidence Interval is certainly no larger. At the discretion of the survey team, it may be **preferable** to use this level (99%) **either**:

      - when a large number of values are being reported concurrently so that some might be expected to appear significant by chance, or

      - when the consequences of erroneous results are likely to be serious.

Statistical Significance - Normal Level to be 5%

11.   The advice on statistical significance is similar to that for Confidence Intervals.

12.   Where there is a choice, confidence intervals or limits are preferred to statistical significance. If two values are to be compared and their confidence intervals do not overlap, there is little need to perform some test of significance (eg Student's t). However, in order to test a comparison between two values, the statistical significance should be evaluated if their Confidence Intervals overlap.

13.   In general, a test of an alternative hypothesis (that true values are different) will be considered statistically significant if the estimated probability of the observed outcome under the null hypothesis (that true values are the same) is less than **5%.**

14.   **One-sided** tests of significance should use a level of **2.5%** (eg is B > A?).

15.   Actual estimates of probability **(p)** may be reported if available. For example, for a one-sided test, a Student's t-value can be compared with a standard value t $_{0.025}$ found in a Statistical Table for **p** = 0.025. However, the table may also provide a good estimate (eg 0.017) for **p** for the particular t-value being assessed. In that case, a significant result may be indicated:

      either by   (p < 0.025) or (p < 2.5%)

      or by   (p = 0.017) or (p = 1.7%).

The latter provides more information but can be more confusing particularly when several results are presented each with their own p-values.

16.   Greater degrees of significance such as **1%** are of course **acceptable** but only **preferable** to 5 or 2.5% at the discretion of the Study Team in circumstances similar to those discussed earlier in paragraph 10.

Sample Size

17.   One of the objectives of a Pilot study must be to discover the amount of inherent and residual **variation** in the population. Once these are known the statistician can recommend minimum desirable sample sizes, provided that the Study Team have identified for which **combinations** of controlled (risk) factors they wish to be able to discriminate between groups. For example, a study needs to be larger if it is to differentiate between old males and young females than if it is to compare old against young or male against female but not the interaction of age and sex effects. It is recommended that the design should aim for **90%** probability of just achieving the required resolving power at the preferred confidence or significance level.

MINIMUM SAMPLE SIZES
FOR GIVEN CONFIDENCE LEVELS/SIGNIFICANCE LEVELS
by required resolution and population standard deviation
(with about 90% power)

Minimum Sample Size at 95% CONFIDENCE LEVEL

	standard deviation		
required resolution	0.5	1.0	1.5
0.1	519	2079	4668
0.3	58	231	519
0.5	21	83	187
1.0	6	21	47

— —

Minimum Sample Size at 99% CONFIDENCE LEVEL

	standard deviation		
required resolution	0.5	1.0	1.5
0.1	733	2929	6590
0.3	82	326	733
0.5	30	118	264
1.0	8	30	66

— —

COST IMPLICATIONS OF SETTING CONFIDENCE LEVELS

1.   Tables appended to the previous paper showed the minimum sample sizes recommended for given levels of confidence, population standard deviation and required resolving power. Although it is possible to develop tables for other confidence levels, there are too many numbers to easily assimilate their meaning. In order to be able to grasp the impact of varying the intended confidence level, it is therefore first necessary to simplify the presentation of the relative sample sizes and their costs.

2.   It is also helpful to identify a particular scenario as the point of reference with which other possibilities are to be compared. Assume therefore that the product under investigation has a population standard deviation (sd) of one unit (in terms of log-10 counts) and that the desired resolving power (rp) is also one unit. The earlier paper showed the minimum sample sizes to be respectively 21 and 30 items for required confidence levels of 95 and 99%. (These were sufficient to allow a power of 90% - ie the chance of achieving the target).

3.   A simple table shows the impact of altering the level of confidence to be assured:

Minimum sample sizes necessary for given confidence levels for standard deviation and resolution of 1 unit

Confidence Level (%)	50	60	70	80	90	95	99
Sample Size*	8	10	11	14	18	21	30
Cost @ £700 + per sample (in £1000)	6	7	8	10	13	15	21

> * These sample sizes should be slightly larger to allow for small sample statistics corrections.
>
> The marginal differences obscure the argument.
> + Estimated costs for EPWG samples.

4.   **It is clear that it roughly trebles the costs involved to improve the assured level of confidence from 50 to 95%, while 50 to 99% means a quadrupling. This rule of thumb holds true for _any_ combination of sd and required rp. That is, whatever the sd and rp, the same approximate factors of three and four still apply.**

5.   Nevertheless it remains that the sd and rp do strongly affect costs. Other things being equal, the minimum sample size is proportional to the square of the ratio of the sd and the rp - ie the ratio multiplied by itself. For example the same sample sizes and costs ensue for sd and rp both equal to 0.3, since their ratio is still one. If however, the sd and desired rp are 1 and 0.3 respectively, all the sample sizes and costs in the above table are increased by a factor of about 11 since their ratio is now about 3.3.

6.   For a given sample size (and cost) it is always possible either:

- to calculate a confidence interval at _any_ desired level, but the resolution may be unacceptably coarse, or

- to allow almost any size of resolution, but the power to identify significant differences may be compromised.

That is, there is potentially a trade-off between sample size (and cost), confidence (or significance) levels, population standard deviation and resolving power.

MINIMUM RECOMMENDED SAMPLE SIZE NECESSARY FOR GIVEN CONFIDENCE LEVEL BY VARYING RELATIVE RESOLUTION (at approximately 90% power)

RESOLUTION

CONF (%)	1.0	0.5	0.3	0.1
50	8	31	86	766
60	10	37	101	902
70	11	43	120	1075
80	14	53	146	1314
90	18	69	191	1713
95	21	85	234	2102
99	30	120	331	2976

RELATIVE RESOLUTION: THE RATIO OF RESOLVING POWER TO STANDARD DEVIATION.

7.   In practice, it must be recognised that considerably more items need to be sampled if a number of 'effects' are to be assessed and compared, such as type of producer and type of product.

AN EXAMPLE OF SAMPLING METHODS ENDORSED BY THE RWG

STUDY OF POTENTIAL CONTAMINATION SITES IN CATERING PREMISES (RETAIL, CATERING AND CONSUMER SURVEILLANCE WORKING GROUP)

Sampling Methods

Method 1 - Cotton Wool Swab technique

A cotton wool swab* technique for sampling reproducible areas of flat or complex-shaped hard surfaces, based on established techniques. A known area of the test surface is swabbed using a sterile aluminium template (Figure 1). The swab heads are broken off into a known volume of recovery fluid and transported to the laboratory.

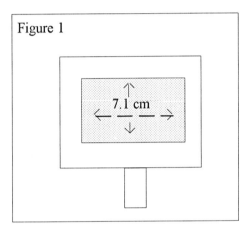

Figure 1

7.1 cm

Equipment

Maximum Recovery Diluent (MRD)   + 0.3% sodium thiosulphite
                                    + 3.0% 'Tween 80' in 10ml screw
                                    capped bottles

Sterile 25cm² templates
Sterile cotton wool swabs
Alcohol impregnated cleaning swabs
Labels

* as referenced in the American Public Health Association
Compendium of Methods for the Microbiological Examination of Foods

Procedure

1. Moisten cotton wool swab in 10ml bottle of supplemented MRD.

2. Place template (see Fig. 1) over area to be swabbed, if this is sufficiently flat. Where the shape of the target surface prevents use of a template, estimate $25cm^2$ as the test area.

3. Rub moistened swab over test area with a twirling motion.

4. Break swab head off into 10ml supplemented MRD.

5. Repeat steps 2 to 4 using a dry sterile swab.

6. Cap the bottle securely, label with sample description and identification number, and place in cool box for transport to the laboratory.

Method 2 - Wash technique

A method for eluting cloths or items with convoluted surfaces eg balloon whisks, so as to obtain a microbiological sample in the eluate. The technique will consist of shaking the item in a sterile bag with diluent and sampling the eluate thus produced.

Equipment

Maximum Recovery Diluent (MRD)   + 0.3% sodium thiosulphite
                                        + 3.0% 'Tween 80'
Sterile 1000ml plastic bags, eg. stomacher bags, with seals and labels.

Procedure

1. Place item into sterile bag eg. 1000ml stomacher bag.

2. Add supplemented MRD in sufficient volume to soak the item. This volume will probably need to be 100ml in order to be sufficient for chef's cloths and will have to be established by experiment.

3. Squeeze or gently shake the bagged item to maximise contact with the eluate. For cloths, make sure to produce free fluid in the bottom of the bag.

4. Remove the test item, seal the bag, label the bag with sample description and identification number, and double seal it within another similar bag.

5. Place sealed bag in cool box for transport to laboratory.

Archive Preservation of Samples and Isolates

C.1.Faecal Samples

Introduction

The method is based on those of Crowther[61] and Hudson[62] in which faecal bacteria are preserved qualitatively and quantitatively for extended periods by rapid freezing in a bacteriological nutrient containing glycerol as cryoprotectant (cryo broth). There are some reductions in the total counts and counts of some genera but these are small compared to losses on storage or freezing in the absence of cryoprotectant.

Method

1.	A 20% suspension of faecal sample is made in cryo broth in a 2ml polypropylene vial. The vial is then labelled with the IID Study number using an indelible felt tip marker.

2.	The vial is then snap-frozen in a -70^0C freezer.

3.	Store samples at or below -70^0C and transfer between laboratories on dry ice or in liquid nitrogen.

4.	Store unused vials of cryo broth at room temperature or at 4^0C. Discard after 6-8 months or if obviously contaminated.

Precautions

5.	Avoid spilling cryoprotectant or diluted sample from the vial and check that the cap is screwed tightly.

6.	Freezing in a domestic type freezer (at -20^0C) is not ideal as considerable losses of flora can occur.

Medium

Cryoprotective broth (Cryo broth)

Lab-Lemco powder	10g
Glycerol	100ml
Distilled water	900ml

Adjust to pH 7.3
Fill as 4.5ml in 7ml bijoux bottle or as 50ml in a medical flat
Sterilize by autoclaving at 115^0C for 20 minutes

C.2 Isolates

Introduction

Isolates are to be preserved for long term storage by binding on porous beads in the presence of cryopreservative [63,64,65] prior to freezing at -70℃. Initial preservation will be carried out by the specialist laboratories, who will then refer preserved cultures to CAMR for long term storage.

Method

1. Using a permanent marker, code a suitable vial containing coloured beads and cryopreservative fluid* with the IID Study number for the sample.
Note. *The 'Microbank' system (available from Pro-Lab Diagnostics) is a commercially available archiving system which has proved suitable for this purpose.

2. Pick a selection of 5 colonies of a young (18-24 hours) typed pure culture growing on nonselective agar for mixed inoculation into the fluid in the vial. Inoculate the fluid to approximately 3-4 Macfarlane standard.

3. Close the vial tightly and invert 4-5 times to mix the contents **without vortexing.**

4. Decant off the fluid leaving the beads as free of liquid as possible. Reclose the vial finger-tight.

5. Freeze the inoculated vial at -70℃ and send to CAMR under suitable conditions to maintain this temperature, e.g. in ice or liquid nitrogen.

Precautions

6. Ensure aseptic conditions to maintain the culture's microbiological purity, while taking care to avoid creating a biohazard from heavy cultures of known pathogens. A microbiological safety cabinet should be used for manipulation of concentrated suspensions, particularly for decanting of inoculated fluid from beads.

7. Vials should not be used if they show any evidence of leakage or loss of fluid; if there is any visible turbidity in the fluid; or if the expiry date on commercially available vials has passed.

References

61 Crowther JC. Transport and storage of faeces for bacterial examination J Appl Bacteriol 1971;34:477-483

62 Hudson, MJ. HIll MJ, Elliott PR, Berghouse LM, Burnham WR, et al, The microbial flora of the rectal mucosa and faeces of patients with Crohn's disease before and during antimicrobial chemotherapy. J Med Microbiol 1984;18:335-345

63 White DJ, Sands RL. Storage of bacteria at -76℃ Medical Laboratory Sciences, 1985;42:289-290

64 Feltham RKA, Power AK, Pell PA, Sneath PHA. A simple method for storage of bacteria at -76℃ J Appl Bacteriol, 1978;44:313-316

65 Nagel JG, Cunz LJ. Simplified storage and retrieval of stock cultures Applied Microbiology 1971;23(4):837-838

GLOSSARY

Aetiology
The cause of a specific disease.

Bacteriophage typing
A method for distinguishing varieties of bacteria ('phage types) within a particular species on the basis of their susceptibilities to a range of bacteriophages (bacterial viruses).

Campylobacter
A Gram negative non-sporing bacterium

Campylobacteriosis
Name of a disease caused by *Campylobacter* species.

Case
A person in the population identified as having a particular disease.

Case control study

An epidemiological study in which the characteristics of persons with a specified disease are compared with a suitable control group of persons without the disease.

Cohort study
An epidemiological study in which a designated group or cohort of people are studied over a period of time to determine their experience of disease and identify possible factors that may influence the occurrence of disease. A cohort study is sometimes referred to as a follow-up longitudinal or prospective study.

Epidemiology
The study of factors affecting health and disease in populations and the application of this study to the control and prevention of disease.

Escherichia coli
A Gram negative non-sporing bacterium.

Food poisoning
Any disease of an infectious or toxic nature caused by or thought to be caused by the consumption of food or water. Food poisoning is a notifiable disease under the Public Health (Control of Disease) Act 1984; Public Health (Infectious Disease) Regulation 1988.

Food poisoning - formal notifications
These are made by a medical practicer (usually a GP) who has a statutory responsibility to report to the Proper Officer who reports weekly to the Registrar General at the Office of Population Censuses and Surveys (OPCS).

Food poisoning - notifications ascertained by other means
If during an investigation of a food poisoning incident further cases emerge, which have not been formally notified, these are also reported to the OPCS as "ascertained by others means".

Haemolytic uraemic syndrome (HUS)
This syndrome may arise from a variety of causes and is characterised by anaemia and kidney failure.

Haemorrhagic colitis
Inflammation and bleeding from the large bowel that may be caused by an infectious agent.

Isolate
A single species of a micro-organism originating from a particular sample (eg faecal isolate) growing in a pure culture.

Jarman deprivation score
A composite measure of factors affecting GP workload.

Laboratory reports
Data routinely collected nationally of laboratory identifications of certain pathogenic organisms. Includes all those known to cause foodborne infections.

Listeria
A Gram positive non-sporing bacterium.

Listeriosis
Disease usually caused by *Listeria monocytogenes*.

Proper Officer (for infectious diseases)
The nominated officer of the relevant local authority. (In England usually the consultant in communicable disease control (CCDC) and in Scotland to the Chief Medical Officer of the health board).

Salmonella
A Gram negative non-sporing bacterium.

Salmonellosis
Infectious Intestinal disease caused by *Salmonella* species.

Serotyping
A method of distinguishing varieties of bacteria (serotypes) by defining their antigenic properties on the basis of their reaction to known antisera. A number of serotypes may constitute a serogroup.

Species
A classification of organisms within a genus which have similarities and can be further subdivided into sub-species.

Sub-species
A classification of organisms within a species which have similarities.

Verocytotoxin producing *Escherichia coli* (VTEC)
A particular sub-species of *E. coli* often of the serogroup O157 which is associated with haemorrhagic colitis and haemolytic uraemic syndrome.

References

[1] Steering Group on the Microbiological Safety of Food: First Report of Progress 1990-1992. ISBN 0-11-321665-3

[2] Steering Group on the Microbiological Safety of Food: Annual Report 1993. ISBN 0-11-321-817-6

Printed in the United Kingdom for HMSO
Dd301406 9/95 C6 G3397 10170